C000144134

# DIABETES AND LAB( ---
# MEDICINE

## Janet Smith B.Sc., M.Sc., MRCPath
Consultant Clinical Biochemist and Hon Senior Lecturer, University Hospital Birmingham NHS Trust, Birmingham, UK

## Malcolm Nattrass B.Sc., M.D., FRCP, FRCPath
Consultant Physician and Hon Senior Lecturer, Selly Oak Hospital, Birmingham, UK

Editors:
William Marshall, FRCP, FRCPath, FRCPEdin, FIBiol
Reader in Clinical Biochemistry, King's College Hospital, London, UK

Janet Horner, B.Sc., MBChB, MRCP, MRCGP, MRCPath
Consultant Chemical Pathologist, St James' University Hospital, Leeds, UK

## ACB VENTURE PUBLICATIONS

Production of this educational publication has been made possible by the generous sponsorship of A.Menarini Diagnostics Ltd and Olympus Diagnostic Systems

ACB VENTURE PUBLICATIONS
Chairman - Mike Hallworth

British Library Cataloguing in Publication Data

A catalogue record for the book is available from the British Library

ISBN 0 902429 31 0 ACB Venture Publications

Cover design by Alan Sherwood of burntcanvasdesign, Kent, www.burntcan-vasdesign.btinternet.co.uk

Layout and typesetting by Roy Sherwood and Emma Davies in Palatino.

Printed by KSC Printers, Tunbridge Wells, Kent

# Preface

It can be argued that diabetes mellitus is the disease that best demonstrates the interrelationship between biochemistry and metabolic medicine. The need for close collaboration between the medical laboratory and the clinical team is exemplified in the diagnosis and management of people with the disorder.

The consequences of an absolute or relative deficiency of insulin profoundly affect intermediary metabolism, leading to acute metabolic crises and long-term medical complications.

The aim of this book is to explore the role of the laboratory in the diagnosis and management of diabetes and its complications, as well as to explain the fundamental changes to biochemical pathways and how these are manifested clinically. Actual clinical cases are incorporated to illustrate these. Most of these were collected during the 1990s when fructosamine, rather than $HbA_{1c}$, was used in our clinic to monitor glycaemic control. To maintain authenticity, we have retained the fructosamine values in the case descriptions but emphasise here that, in 2004, $HbA_{1c}$ should be used as the index of glycaemic control, as recommended by the United Kingdom National Service Frameworks for Diabetes Mellitus and national and international advisory bodies.

We are indebted to the following colleagues who were mainly responsible for writing the following chapters: Dr Fidema Dunne - Pregnancy and diabetes; Dr Jonathan Webber - Hyperglycaemic comas and Dr Andrew Willis - Complications of diabetes, and also to Drs Andrew Hartland and Jyoti Sidhu, who identified and prepared the clinical cases.

We would also like to thank all the staff of the Diabetes Centre and Clinical Biochemistry departments at Selly Oak Hospital who together enable us to provide our collaborative diabetes clinic service to South Birmingham.

Finally, we thank ACB Venture Publications for inviting us to write this book and in particular our editors Drs William Marshall and Janet Horner, Dr Roy Sherwood for the design and layout of the book and Beverley Harris for proof-reading.

Malcolm Nattrass
Janet Smith
April 2004

# ACKNOWLEDGEMENTS

The authors are grateful to the following for permission to reproduce or adapt material for certain figures used in this publication:

Annals of Clinical Biochemistry 2000; 37: 588-592 (Fig 3.2)

**Important notice**

Although ACB Venture Publications has made every effort to ensure the accuracy of the information contained in this book, the responsibility for the patient is ultimately that of the medical practitioner ordering or performing/supervising the investigations. All drugs and intravenous fluids must be prescribed by a registered medical practitioner and administered by an individual authorised to do so. The publishers, authors and editors do not assume any liability for any injury and/or damage to persons or property arising from this publication.

# Contents

# Chapter 1

# The Aetiology of Diabetes

## INTRODUCTION

Diabetes mellitus is a chronic metabolic disorder characterised by a tendency to hyperglycaemia and to the development of atherosclerosis, retinopathy, neuropathy and nephropathy. It is a major risk factor for coronary heart disease. In most patients, diabetes is primary and is classified as either type 1 or type 2, but diabetes can also occur secondarily to other conditions, notably pancreatic and some endocrine diseases.

## TYPE 1 DIABETES

Type 1 diabetes typically has an abrupt onset with thirst, polyuria, and weight loss. Hyperglycaemia may be accompanied by ketonuria and ketoacidosis. The underlying defect is insulin deficiency. Although the clinical onset is usually sudden, in some individuals there is evidence of a long subclinical period. Type 1 diabetes is generally considered to be an autoimmune disease, with both genetic and environmental precipitating factors contributing to its pathogenesis.

## GENETIC FACTORS

It has been recognised for many years that type 1 diabetes has a substantial genetic component to its aetiology. However, no single gene has been identified that predicts diabetes although a number of significant links have emerged, particularly with the major histocompatibility system and the insulin gene.

### THE MAJOR HISTOCOMPATIBILITY SYSTEM

The major contribution to the genetic tendency in type 1 diabetes lies in the human leukocyte antigens (HLA) of the major histocompatibility system. Genes encoding these antigens, which are present on all nucleated cell surfaces (HLA A, B, C: Class I) or on some cells only (HLA D, DR: Class II), are located on the short arm of chromosome 6. This location is close to genes that influence the immunological response, including antibody production and cell mediated immunity.

The HLA system is highly polymorphic, with each locus encoding a different cell surface antigen. Current evidence points to a significant increase in relative risk of developing type 1 diabetes with specific HLA antigens. The strongest associations in a Caucasian population are between the disease and HLA DR3 and DR4, while there is a negative association with HLA DR2. About 90% of Caucasian patients with type 1 diabetes are positive for DR3 or DR4. DR3 and DR4 confer additive risk such that

1

the heterozygote genotype DR3/DR4 shows an increased relative risk, even over the homozygotes.

HLA-DR antigens are made up of two A-chains and two B-chains. Other Class II antigens, distinct from the DR antigen, are the DQ antigens, which are in strong linkage disequilibrium with DR and the DP antigens. The DQ region is composed of two α genes, DQA1 and DQA2, and two β genes, DQB1 and DQB2. Studies have identified certain amino acid sequences in DQ regions with links to type 1 diabetes. Thus aspartate at position 57 of the DQB1 chain appears to confer resistance to type 1 diabetes, while arginine at position 52 in the DQA1 chain results in susceptibility.

*POLYMORPHISM OF THE INSULIN GENE*
The insulin gene resides on the short arm of chromosome 11. Genetic polymorphism of the 5′ flanking region of the human insulin gene has been found. This polymorphism is due to a region of variable number of tandem repeats (VNTR). The three alleles identified are simply classed as 1, 2 or 3 and of these, the class 2 allele is exceedingly rare. The class 1 allele, with 50 repeats, predisposes to type 1 diabetes, while the class 3 allele, with 150-200 repeats, is protective.

*OTHER SUSCEPTIBILITY GENES*
It is clear that the genetic component cannot be accounted for in its entirety by a contribution from HLA antigens and the insulin gene. In quantitative terms, the HLA system probably accounts for around 40% of susceptibility and the insulin gene around 10%. In searches of the human genome, a number of other linkages have been identified, particularly on chromosomes 11q and 6q. It can be safely assumed that no other strong genetic links will be identified and any remaining linkages are likely to contribute less than 6% each. Thus the unidentified genetic component of type 1 diabetes is likely to comprise many different loci.

ENVIRONMENTAL FACTORS
Environmental factors play a major part in precipitating overt disease. The main factors that have been identified as having potential for precipitating type 1 diabetes are viruses and chemical toxins.

*VIRUSES*
The evidence to implicate viruses in the aetiology of type 1 diabetes comes from population studies, animal experiments and some limited human information. In population studies, the main association is between mumps infection and type 1 diabetes. Epidemics of mumps that occurred in the past were clearly followed by an 'outbreak' of type 1 diabetes.

It is clear from data on the incidence of type 1 diabetes that there is a seasonal incidence, as well as peaks of incidence at specific ages. It has been argued that both the seasonal and age incidence follow a similar pattern to that of viral infections in children. Furthermore, blood taken from children at the time of diagnosis of diabetes has revealed a higher incidence of antibodies to coxsackievirus B4 than in non-diabetic children.

In mice, a diabetes-like disease can be induced by the M variant of the encephalomyocarditis virus, while in other rodents, reovirus, Group B coxsackievirus and Venezuelan equine encephalitis virus all produce diabetes.

There is an association between type 1 diabetes and congenital rubella, but direct evidence of viral infection of the pancreas has proved elusive. Occasional patients with diabetes who died from overwhelming viral infection have been shown to have viral particles in the pancreas, although whether this has more general relevance is uncertain.

### CHEMICALS
It has been recognised for many years that certain chemicals result in β cell destruction and diabetes, when injected into animals. The best known are alloxan and streptozotocin. In human diabetes, identification of destructive agents is more difficult owing to the vast numbers of chemicals ingested daily. Of interest is the increased incidence of type 1 diabetes in groups that consume large quantities of smoked meat and fish. More recently, epidemiological studies have suggested that prolonged breast feeding protects against the development of diabetes. This has been interpreted as evidence that the introduction of cows' milk protein might increase susceptibility to type 1 diabetes.

## IMMUNOLOGICAL FACTORS
Type 1 diabetes has a well-recognised association with thyroid disease, Addison's disease and pernicious anaemia, and the link between organ specific endocrinopathies and diabetes has been accepted for many years. In the early 1970s, antibodies to islet cells were detected in blood from diabetic patients with other autoimmune disorders; they were also reported in patients with newly-diagnosed type 1 diabetes. They were not specific for particular islet cell types but reacted with all cell types, although not with islet hormones.

These islet cell antibodies may be present for long periods before diabetes becomes clinically overt. Following development and diagnosis of the disease, the majority of patients show a rapid decline in titre (in contrast to the autoantibodies in other autoimmune endocrine diseases) although 10-15% of patients may have persistent antibodies. In this latter group, there is a female preponderance and many patients have evidence of other organ specific antibodies, suggesting a specific sub-group of type 1 diabetes.

Most of the islet cell antibodies are directed against glutamic acid decarboxylase (GAD), an enzyme localised within pancreatic β cells. Isoforms of GAD are also present in inhibitory central nervous system neurones that secrete γ-aminobutyric acid. The rare neurological condition, 'stiff man syndrome', is due to autoimmune destruction of these neurones. Patients with this condition also have islet cell antibodies, consistent with GAD being the islet cell antigen.

## TYPE 2 DIABETES

In type 2 diabetes there is a broad spectrum of presentation from asymptomatic individuals or moderately symptomatic individuals (the majority), to acutely ill patients with considerable metabolic abnormality, who may be in coma. Many patients have clearly had the disease for some years before diagnosis and about 20% of newly diagnosed type 2 diabetic patients have evidence of long term complications at diagnosis. The variety of presentations may support the view that type 2 diabetes is not a homogeneous entity although, with the exception of certain subsets of the condition, this view has coloured the approach to elucidating the aetiology.

## GENETIC FACTORS

The strongest evidence of a genetic influence in the aetiology of type 2 diabetes comes from studies in identical twins, which have shown that the concordance rate is of the order of 90%. This contrasts with the 45-50% concordance rate for type 1 diabetes, despite this disease also having a clear genetic component. In family studies, about 40% of siblings of patients with type 2 diabetes will become diabetic before the age of 80 years.

### CANDIDATE GENES

Despite this apparently strong genetic component, there is only limited information on the likely genetic markers. No strong associations have been found in Caucasian populations with particular HLA antigens, nor has an association been identified with the genes that encode for insulin or the insulin receptor.

## ENVIRONMENTAL FACTORS

Environmental precipitants are almost as elusive. Age, diet, obesity, exercise and stress have all been suggested but, while it is true that type 2 diabetes becomes more common with increasing age, and that obesity is regularly observed in patients in the diabetes clinic, these observations hardly contribute to our understanding of aetiology. A rise in the concentrations of catabolic hormones can clearly precipitate diabetes in patients who are predisposed and this is commonly seen accompanying a myocardial infarction. The relationship of this stress to the layman's version of stress is unclear, but it seems unlikely that the stress of day-to-day living can precipitate diabetes.

Undoubtedly, a change in life-style from active to more sedentary may unmask a genetic predisposition to diabetes, as has occurred in specific populations such as the Pima Indians of Arizona and the Nauruans. While reduced physical activity may be implicated, however, it is difficult to divorce from change in diet and obesity.

Diabetes may follow accidental trauma, but whether this is the onset of disease is dubious. It is quite common to be asked whether diabetes, first detected after an accident, was caused by the accident. It is more usual to consider the injury as unmasking previously present but undetected diabetes or providing an opportunity for fortuitous diagnosis through 'routine' testing of blood or urine.

Hales and colleagues have argued that fetal and early life nutrition are important determinants for the later development of impaired glucose tolerance and type 2 diabetes. They studied men in their sixties whose weights in early life were known. A clear relationship emerged between low birth weight and low weight at twelve months with abnormal glucose tolerance in later life. On the basis of these data, it has been suggested that early (including those occurring *in utero*) nutritional factors that determine fetal and infant growth influence the size and vascularity of the adult pancreas. Combined in later life with obesity, inactivity or ageing resulting in insulin resistance, this could lead to the development of glucose intolerance.

It is worth drawing attention to the different habitus which obesity can take in individuals, the 'apples and pears' debate. The pear-shaped form of the human carrying excess fat predominantly around the buttocks and thighs may be less harmful in its consequences than the apple shape, where fat is carried predominantly as an intra-abdominal apron. In practical terms, waist:hip ratio may be a more potent predictor of cardiovascular outcome in obese patients than the body mass index.

## SECONDARY DIABETES

## PANCREATIC DISEASE

### PANCREATITIS
Hyperglycaemia is common during an attack of acute pancreatitis and may mark the onset of diabetes, but this is uncommon. It is thought that an inflammatory lesion severe enough to destroy more than 85% of the islets would probably be fatal.

Certainly, in chronic pancreatitis, diabetes only appears after a significant proportion of the gland has been destroyed.

In chronic pancreatitis, about one-third of patients subsequently develop diabetes and one-third impaired glucose tolerance, although this is not an important numerical cause of diabetes in Europe or North America. There is considerable geographic disparity in diabetes secondary to chronic pancreatitis, probably reflecting different aetiologies. In the Western world, alcohol is the clearest precipitating cause.

There is marked variation in insulin responses to oral glucose and subnormal, normal, and supranormal responses are reported. Islet cell antibodies are not present.

The histological changes vary. Islet preservation has been reported even when exocrine destruction is severe. Islet clustering, or a decrease in the number of islets may be present. Some islets show degeneration and round cell infiltration. With increasing hyalinisation of fibrous tissue, the islets are distorted into linear streaks. Immunocytochemistry suggests that B cell numbers are reduced and those of A cells increased, sometimes to equal the total number of B cells, with normal numbers of D cells and a slight increase in PP cells.

### CARCINOMA OF THE PANCREAS

Diabetes mellitus is a recognised (albeit uncommon) presentation of carcinoma of the pancreas. The story is usually typical, with little to suggest an underlying neoplasm when the patient is first seen. Weight loss is usually a presenting feature, but is ascribed to diabetes. With treatment the hyperglycaemia settles, glycosuria, and hence loss of energy, resolves, but weight is not regained or loss continues. It is often not until the appearance of painless jaundice or back pain that the cause of the weight loss becomes apparent.

A mysterious feature of the diabetes associated with carcinoma of the pancreas is that islet cell destruction by the growth or associated pancreatitis is often not extensive and a considerable part of the gland may appear normal on routine examination.

### TOTAL PANCREATECTOMY

Complete pancreatectomy leads inevitably to diabetes that does not respond to sulphonylurea drugs and which requires insulin treatment. Withdrawal of insulin leads rapidly to osmotic symptoms and, usually, ketosis, although some patients do not develop ketosis, presumably because of the lack of pancreatic glucagon. The daily requirement of insulin is usually small, commonly of the order of 10 to 20 units, which is less than the average for type 1 diabetes. The reason for this is uncertain. It may be lack of glucagon but it may also be changes in absorption of nutrients in the gut as a consequence of loss of exocrine function.

HAEMOCHROMATOSIS
In haemochromatosis, the iron content of the pancreas is increased 50-100 times normal and the end result is extensive pancreatic fibrosis. Islets, which may be reduced in number or even absent, are pigmented in 80% of cases, and pigment may also be deposited in the acinar or ductal tissues. It may be sufficient to colour the pancreas reddish brown. The involvement of the islets may not be uniform, with β cells preferentially affected and the α cells remaining quantitatively normal. It is commonly held that diabetes accompanying haemochromatosis results from this iron deposition.

The diabetes of haemochromatosis is not obviously different to other types of diabetes and most patients end up on insulin treatment. It has been suggested that control of diabetes may improve with chelation therapy, which may be through an effect on the pancreas, although it is possible that it is due to an improvement in liver function.

Haemochromatosis is a rare cause of diabetes, occurring in less than 1% of diabetic patients. The old description of it as 'bronze diabetes' is not always apt. The pigmentation may be grey (metallic) rather than bronze (melanotic) and may not be recognised. Enlargement of the liver at presentation calls for investigation, especially if the skin has an unusual colour. Estimation of the serum iron and iron binding capacity, with calculation of the percentage saturation of transferrin, is a useful screening procedure, although serum ferritin measurement provides a more specific assessment of iron stores. Liver biopsy should be confirmatory but there is often difficulty in deciding whether haemochromatosis or haemosiderosis is the underlying lesion. If in doubt about the diagnosis, demonstration that the absorption of radioactive iron from the gut is abnormal is diagnostic of haemochromatosis.

It is now known that in Caucasians, haemochromatosis is associated with mutations in the HFE gene. Two amino acid substitutions, C282Y and H63D, have been identified, with most affected subjects being either homozygous for the C282Y mutation or compound heterozygotes. Genetic tests based on the polymerase chain reaction and restriction enzyme digests are now available and have largely replaced liver biopsy and the radiolabelled iron absorption test in the diagnosis of haemochromatosis. In non-Caucasian subjects, however, these mutations are rare and the iron accumulation may be due to overexposure to iron, although new genes have recently been found that are implicated in iron metabolism (the IReg genes) and these may account for the excess iron absorption.

## MALNUTRITION-RELATED DIABETES

Malnutrition-related diabetes is an important cause of diabetes worldwide. For example, it accounts for 7% of diabetes in Jamaica, 23% in India and according to some reports, 80% of diabetes in Indonesia. The syndrome is also known as J-type diabetes, Z-type diabetes, tropical diabetes, tropical calcific pancreatitis, fibrocalculous diabetes and protein deficient diabetes. There are two major subtypes, fibrocalculous pancreatic diabetes (also known as tropical calcific pancreatitis) and protein-deficient pancreatic diabetes.

The diagnostic criteria for patients with protein-deficient pancreatic diabetes include onset before the age of 30 years with a history of childhood malnutrition or poor socioeconomic status. Patients should be thin (BMI < 19 kg/m$^2$) with an insulin requirement of greater than 60 units/day or 1.5 units/kg, and if insulin is withdrawn there should be no development of ketoacidosis.

The diagnostic criteria for fibrocalculous pancreatic diabetes are similar, but in addition there should be a history of chronic pancreatitis. Evidence of this is accepted if there are pancreatic calculi. Where these are not obvious, a history of recurrent abdominal pain from an early age, steatorrhoea, an abnormal pancreatic CT scan or ERCP, or an abnormal pancreatic exocrine function test may establish the diagnosis.

The clinical presentation is often with severe diabetes, marked hyperglycaemia and dehydration in an emaciated patient. Patients are underweight yet, by definition, ketosis is absent. The reason for this is unclear. There may be sufficient residual β cell secretion to inhibit hepatic ketogenesis; damage to the α cells may result in the loss of the ketogenic effect of glucagon, or there may be hepatic carnitine deficiency. Alternatively, subcutaneous fat loss may lead to a poor supply of non-esterified fatty acids to the liver for ketogenesis or the action of catecholamines upon lipolysis may be impaired. The response to oral hypoglycaemic agents is poor and large doses of insulin are required to control the blood glucose.

Malnutrition, with or without cassava consumption, is thought to play a role in the aetiology of this condition. Cassava intake is high in many areas where this type of diabetes occurs. It contains linamarin, a glycoside that on hydrolysis releases hydrocyanic acid. This is normally inactivated by conjugation with the sulphydryl groups of the amino acids methionine, cystine, and cysteine, which are deficient in protein calorie malnutrition. There are areas where malnutrition-related diabetes is endemic and cassava is the main staple food, but there are other areas where the syndrome is common yet the intake of cassava is low. Currently the link remains non proven.

# DRUGS

It is often difficult to state with any certainty that a particular drug or class of drugs causes hyperglycaemia or diabetes. The appearance of diabetes after the use of a particular drug may simply be an indication of a diabetic predisposition with the onset having been unmasked by the drug. Having said that, however, it is clear that the administration of some drugs has a clearly detrimental effect upon diabetic control in patients with established diabetes.

## THIAZIDE DIURETICS

Hyperglycaemia after taking thiazide diuretics has been known for some time. The effect is especially striking in the case of the antihypertensive agent, diazoxide. Since the effect was observed, diazoxide has probably been used as much in the treatment of non-diabetic hypoglycaemia as it has as an antihypertensive agent.

During thiazide treatment, plasma insulin concentrations in response to secretogogues are reduced. This is likely to be the result of potassium depletion, which impairs insulin secretion. Hyperglycaemia appears within a variable time from a few days to many months after starting treatment. It is usually relatively moderate and may disappear if the drug is withdrawn. In some instances, the diabetes does not seem to be reversible. The response to a sulphonylurea is excellent.

## ANTIHYPERTENSIVE AGENTS

Other antihypertensive agents have been reported to alter glucose homeostasis. The most important of these are beta-blockers. A number of studies have shown that propranolol can result in glucose intolerance in previously non-diabetic patients, although the effect is small and of doubtful clinical significance. The mechanism whereby beta-blockers cause glucose intolerance is unclear.

## ADRENERGIC BETA-AGONISTS

Adrenergic beta$_2$-agonists are widely used in the treatment of bronchial asthma but it was their use in premature labour that lead to reports of effects upon glucose homeostasis. Salbutamol, terbutaline and ritodrine have all been shown to raise blood glucose and lactate concentrations, and to induce hypokalaemia. A metabolic acidosis may accompany these abnormalities. The mechanism is unclear, although the raised glucose is accompanied by raised circulating insulin.

## CORTICOSTEROIDS

Corticosteroid preparations are potent precipitators of overt diabetes and cause loss of control in established diabetic patients when given in large doses. The mechanism by which this is brought about is considered below.

*OTHER DRUGS*

The other major group of drugs, which has attracted particular interest, is the immunosuppressive agents. The development of diabetes or impaired glucose tolerance in post-transplant patients receiving immunosuppressive agents is common. The effect is not due solely to concomitant administration of corticosteroids, since it persists after discontinuing steroids. Nor is it due to severe insulinopenia: it may result from insulin resistance with or without a subtle impairment of insulin secretion.

## ENDOCRINE DISEASE

*CUSHING'S SYNDROME*

Corticosteroids are potent antagonists of insulin, with effects on carbohydrate, protein and fat metabolism, and it is not surprising, therefore, that excessive secretion of corticosteroids has long been associated with diabetes. Approximately two-thirds of patients with Cushing's syndrome have abnormalities of glucose tolerance.

Steroids increase fasting blood glucose concentrations but with more prolonged corticosteroid excess, glucose intolerance develops although blood glucose may return to normal. The increase in blood glucose concentrations is due to stimulation of hepatic gluconeogenesis through an effect upon key enzymes such as phosphoenolpyruvate carboxykinase. Supply of gluconeogenic precursors is also increased. Cortisol also inhibits insulin-stimulated glucose uptake into muscle and adipose tissue. In insulin deficiency, ketone body concentrations are elevated by cortisol excess.

Attention should be drawn to the association of diabetes with the ectopic ACTH syndrome. At presentation, there is a history of weight loss and weakness. Both may be severe, the former suggesting type 1 diabetes; the latter is due more to hypokalaemia than diabetes. Pigmentation of the palms and other sites is usually obvious. The prognosis is poor.

*ACROMEGALY*

Growth hormone increases hepatic glucose output and impairs peripheral glucose uptake, but if diabetes occurs in patients with acromegaly, it is usually biochemically mild. Growth hormone also has a lipolytic effect, which results in increased ketone body concentrations.

In all endocrine diseases where the action of insulin is antagonised by another hormone, it has been suggested that there is a progression to diabetes. This starts with normal glucose tolerance associated with hyperinsulinaemia, and progresses through impaired glucose tolerance despite hyperinsulinaemia to diabetes with insulin deficiency. However, only 5-10% of acromegalic patients develop frank diabetes.

### PHAEOCHROMOCYTOMA

Phaeochromocytoma is a rare endocrine tumour, usually diagnosed during the investigation of hypertension. Diabetes may be present in about 10% of patients with this condition and a further 10% have other abnormalities of glucose tolerance.

Adrenaline inhibits insulin secretion through an alpha-adrenergic effect, and catecholamines are potent inducers of insulin resistance. A prime metabolic effect of catecholamines is to increase hepatic glucose output. This is achieved by both stimulation of glycogen breakdown and an increase in hepatic gluconeogenesis. In the periphery, catecholamines are potent lipolytic agents through increased activity of hormone-sensitive lipase.

Fasting blood glucose concentrations tend to be normal in patients with phaeochromocytoma although the response to oral glucose is impaired. Alpha-adrenergic blockade may restore glucose tolerance to normal, as may resection of the tumour.

### HYPERALDOSTERONISM

Primary hyperaldosteronism is associated with glucose intolerance in about 50% of cases. The biochemical disorder is mild. It seems unlikely that the association is a result of a weak glucocorticoid effect of aldosterone and more likely that it is produced by the hypokalaemia induced by this hormone. Glucose intolerance is also a feature of hypokalaemic hepatic cirrhosis associated with secondary aldosteronism and in both primary and secondary hyperaldosteronism, glucose intolerance may be corrected by repletion of total body potassium stores. The glucose intolerance of Conn's syndrome is also corrected by removal of the adenoma.

### PANCREATIC ENDOCRINE TUMOURS

### Glucagonoma

The clinical syndrome associated with a glucagon secreting tumour comprises weight loss, a normochromic normocytic anaemia, stomatitis, glucose intolerance and markedly elevated concentrations of circulating glucagon. There is often a specific skin rash on the lower legs called necrolytic migratory erythema. The effect of the massive elevations in glucagon upon glucose tolerance is perhaps easier to understand than the other clinical features produced.

Glucagon has potent metabolic effects, increasing glycogen breakdown and gluco-neogenesis, and promoting ketogenesis. It has no effect upon lipolysis in man in physiological concentrations. The effect upon ketogenesis is therefore independent of an effect upon fatty acid availability and is truly intrahepatic.

Glucose intolerance in the glucagonoma syndrome varies in reports from mild to uncontrollable. Since the majority of tumours are malignant, complete resection is rarely possible and glucose intolerance persists.

*Somatostatinoma*
This is a tumour of pancreatic D cells. The most frequent presentation is with gall-stones. Other commonly associated features are dyspepsia, diarrhoea and weight loss. Somatostatin is a potent inhibitor of insulin and glucagon secretion and it is therefore not surprising that diabetes is associated with somatostatinoma. Interestingly, although the diabetes is associated with hypoinsulinaemia, patients with this condition do not appear to be ketosis-prone. As with glucagonomas, the majority of somatostatinomas are malignant.

SYNDROMES OF DIABETES (*See Figure 1.1*)

*DIDMOAD*
The DIDMOAD syndrome (diabetes insipidus, diabetes mellitus, optic atrophy leading to blindness, and deafness) is rare. Presentation is in childhood. The diabetes mellitus is insulin-dependent and shows a tendency to the development of ketoacid-osis. Diabetes insipidus is usually insidious in onset and there is a temptation to blame poor diabetic control for the thirst and polyuria. Deafness often passes un-noticed without objective testing. Other abnormalities have been noted as part of the syndrome, including ataxia and psychiatric disorder, cardiomyopathy, hypo-gonadism, sideroblastic anaemia and thrombocytopoenia.

*MATERNALLY INHERITED DIABETES AND DEAFNESS*
For many years, it has been apparent that there is a maternal effect in the inheritance of diabetes, thus raising the possibility that mitochondrial DNA may play a part in the transmission. A number of groups have reported families with maternal trans-mission of predominantly type 2 diabetes associated with a sensorineural deafness. These patients have a point mutation in their mitochondrial DNA at position 3243 in the mitochondrial tRNA$^{LEU(UUR)}$ gene. This same mutation is responsible for the MELAS syndrome of myopathy, encephalopathy, lactic acidosis, and stroke-like episodes.

## MATURITY ONSET DIABETES OF THE YOUNG (MODY)

Maturity onset diabetes of the young (MODY) has received much attention recently. It would appear to be a heterogeneous collection of genetic causes of diabetes. In the original description, MODY was a syndrome of biochemically mild, sometimes even asymptomatic, diabetes, affecting children, adolescents or young adults. The strong familial segregation of this type of diabetes was recognised soon after the original description. Much later, attention was drawn to the long natural history and only minimal diabetic complications. This description has been extended to include any familial diabetes where some young affected relatives are identified by glucose tolerance tests. A lack of complications is not a feature in some cases and the biochemical disorder may be more severe than in the original description, with some patients requiring insulin.

A number of genetic markers have been identified that feature in subsets of the MODY syndrome. The commonest, which produces a mild biochemical disorder, is an association with mutations of the glucokinase gene. Not all families labelled MODY have glucokinase mutations and even when this mutation is present, genetic heterogeneity exists.

## LIPOATROPHIC DIABETES

In lipoatrophic diabetes, there is total absence of all normal fat depots, diabetes with insulin resistance, hepatomegaly with increased fat storage progressing to fibrosis and cirrhosis, hyperlipidaemia with eruptive xanthomata, and a raised metabolic rate.

The clinical appearance is striking and has been described as cadaveric. The total absence of subcutaneous fat highlights the anatomy of muscles and veins, giving an appearance of muscular hypertrophy. Hyperglycaemia is rarely accompanied by mild ketonaemia but never by ketoacidosis; there is massive insulin resistance.

A congenital form occurs in which parental consanguinity is found. Affected children also manifest growth disorders. Other patients present in later life, although rarely after the age of 30, when onset of lipoatrophy may precede or be simultaneous with onset of diabetes. These cases tend not to be familial and may represent an acquired type of the disease.

Leprechaunism is a severe form of lipoatrophic diabetes. The absence of subcutaneous fat combined with lanugo hair on the face, low-set ears, wide eyes, and thick hair produce the appearance of the leprechaun of Irish mythology. There is a defect in intracellular signalling following insulin's binding to its receptor.

*MENDENHALL SYNDROME*

Mendenhall described a syndrome of short stature with pineal hyperplasia, phallic enlargement, facial dysmorphism, premature dentition and acanthosis nigricans.

Insulin resistant diabetes presents in the first decade and death from ketoacidosis usually occurs in the second decade. Doses of insulin of thousands of units are ineffective; hypophysectomy has been tried with scant success but some patients show a partial response to IGF-1.

*OTHER GENETIC SYNDROMES AND DIABETES*

Since diabetes is a relatively common disease, it has been associated with many genetic syndromes. It is commoner than would be anticipated in Down's, Turner's and Klinefelter's syndromes.

In children, diabetes is associated with the Prader-Willi syndrome of hypotonia, obesity, learning difficulties, and hypogonadotrophic hypogonadism; the Lawrence-Moon-Biedl syndrome of learning difficulty, hypogonadotrophic hypogonadism, retinitis pigmentosa and digital abnormalities, and Alstrom's syndrome of obesity, retinitis pigmentosa and deafness. These syndromes are generally associated with diabetes that does not require insulin for treatment.

In adults, there is an association of diabetes with the neurological diseases dystrophia myotonica, Huntingdon's chorea, and Friedreich's ataxia. In the first two, insulin treatment is not usually required, whereas it may be for diabetes associated with Friedreich's ataxia.

*GENETIC SYNDROMES OF PSEUDO-INSULIN RESISTANCE*

In pseudo-insulin resistance, apparently markedly raised concentrations of insulin accompany normoglycaemia or hyperglycaemia. On investigation, however, the insulin can be shown to be something other than normal human insulin. For example, a mutant insulin secreted as a result of a genetic abnormality may be identified. A similar picture is found in familial hyperproinsulinaemia, in which a genetic defect prevents cleavage of proinsulin to insulin and C-peptide. Large amounts of proinsulin are secreted. Antibodies used in immunoassays show considerable variability in their specificity and may cross react with proinsulin and C-peptide (*see p.154*). In both of these conditions, the response of blood glucose to exogenous insulin is normal.

*SYNDROMES OF INSULIN RESISTANCE AND ACANTHOSIS NIGRICANS*

A number of syndromes have been reported in which massive insulin resistance is associated with acanthosis nigricans. Type A is mainly a syndrome affecting females, presenting before the age of 30, with diabetes or glucose intolerance, severe insulin resistance, acanthosis nigricans and excessive androgen secretion. There is a variable degree of virilisation, with polycystic ovaries, amenorrhoea and moderate elevations in plasma testosterone concentrations. The insulin resistance is to both endogenous and exogenous insulin and is impressive with little effect of doses of insulin as high as 1000 or even 10,000 units. Abnormal insulin binding to its receptor or defective autophosphorylation has been demonstrated.

The type B syndrome has an onset after the age of 30 and is associated with other immunological disease. Anti-nuclear and anti-DNA antibodies may be present, associated with clinical features of systemic lupus erythematosus. The majority of patients (80%) have acanthosis nigricans and all have IgG antibodies directed at the insulin receptor. Occasional variants of both syndromes have been reported. Where the type A syndrome is associated with normal receptors and a post-binding defect, it is known as Type C.

It is unclear whether these syndromes are genetic or acquired. What has become clear is that not all patients with diabetes and acanthosis nigricans have one of these syndromes. Acanthosis nigricans is relatively common among the diabetic population, particularly those of Afro-Caribbean or Asian origin in whom it is unclear whether it signals anything other than an accompaniment to obesity.

## Syndromes associated with diabetes

### Syndromes of insulin resistance

Mendenhall syndrome
> short stature with pineal hyperplasia; facial dysmorphism; phallic enlargement; acanthosis nigricans

Ataxia telangectasia
> insulin resistance; cerebellar ataxia; widespread telangectasia; thymic dysplasia; acanthosis nigricans

Types A, B and C insulin resistance with acanthosis nigricans
> insulin resistance; acanthosis nigricans; virilization

### Lipoatrophic diabetes

Total lipoatrophy
> absence of fat deposits; hepatic enlargement progressing to fibrosis and cirrhosis; hyperlipidaemia with eruptive xanthomata; insulin resistance

Partial lipoatrophy
> as above but with partial loss of fat deposits

Leprechaunism
> absence of subcutaneous fat; lanugo hair on the face; low set ears; wide eyes; thick hair

### Others

Down's syndrome
Turner's syndrome
Klinefelter's syndrome
Prader-Willi syndrome
Lawrence-Moon-Biedl syndrome
Alstrom's syndrome

### Neurological disease

Dystrophia myotonica
Friedrich's ataxia
Huntingdon's chorea

Figure 1.1 Syndromes associated with diabetes

# FURTHER READING

Baekkeskov S, Aanstoot HJ, Christgau S *et al*. Identification of the 64K autoantigen in insulin-dependent diabetes as the GABA-synthesising enzyme glutamic acid decarboxylase. Nature 1990; **347:** 151-6.

Bennett ST, Lucassen AM, Gough SCL *et al*. Susceptibility to human type 1 diabetes at IDDM2 is determined by tandem repeat variation at the insulin gene minisatellite locus. Nat Genet 1995; **9:** 284-91.

Bottazzo GF, Florin-Christensen A, Doniach D. Islet cell antibodies in diabetes mellitus with polyendocrine deficiencies. Lancet 1974; **II:** 1279-83.

Hales CN, Barker DJP, Clark PMS *et al*. Fetal and infant growth and impaired glucose tolerance at age 64. Brit Med J 1991; **303:** 1019-22.

Hattersley AT, Turner RC, Permutt MA *et al*. Linkage of type 2 diabetes to the glucokinase gene. Lancet 1992; **339:** 1307-10.

Krentz AJ, Dousset B, Mayer D *et al*. Metabolic effects of cyclosporin A and FK506 in liver transplant patients. Diabetes 1993; **42:** 1753-9.

Lawrence RD. Lipodystrophy and hepatomegaly with diabetes lipaemia and other metabolic disturbances. Lancet 1946; **I:** 724-31.

Mendenhall EN. Tumour of the pineal body with high insulin resistance. J Indiana Med Assoc 1950; **43:** 32-6.

Neel JV. Diabetes mellitus: a thrifty genotype rendered detrimental by 'progress'. Am J Hum Genet 1962; **14:** 353-62.

Suzuki S, Hinokio Y, Hirai S et al. Pancreatic beta-cell secretory defect associated with the mitochondrial point mutation of the tRNA$^{LEU(UUR)}$ gene: a study in seven families with mitochondrial encephalopathy, lactic acidosis, and stroke-like episodes (MELAS). Diabetologia 1994; **37:** 818-25.

## CLINICAL CASES

### AN UNUSUAL PRESENTATION OF DIABETES IN A MAN

A 62 year old Caucasian man, a lifelong smoker, complained to his family doctor of an exacerbation of his habitual cough. His phlegm was its usual yellow colour but he had noticed a few 'dark brown specks' in it recently. There had been no noticeable weight loss, but his appetite was poor. His only medication was salbutamol and becotide inhalers.

On examination he had palmar pigmentation and a supraclavicular lymph node was palpable. Examination of the respiratory system revealed widespread coarse crackles.

The family doctor took a blood sample for further investigations:

| Analyte (serum) | Result | Reference range |
|---|---|---|
| Sodium (mmol/L) | 144 | 134 -146 |
| Potassium (mmol/L) | 2.7 | 3.4 - 5.2 |
| Urea (mmol/L) | 8.9 | 3.4 - 8.0 |
| Creatinine (µmol/L) | 134 | 60 - 126 |
| Bilirubin (µmol/L) | 21 | 1 - 22 |
| AST (U/L) | 34 | 5 - 43 |
| Alkaline phoshatase (U/L) | 302 | 70 - 330 |
| Albumin (g/L) | 34 | 34 - 51 |
| Glucose (mmol/L) | 15 | |

A chest X-ray showed hilar shadowing and a right lower lobe mass. A provisional diagnosis of carcinoma of the bronchus was made and because of the abnormal biochemical results some further investigations were undertaken. These showed:

| Analyte | Result | Reference range |
| --- | --- | --- |
| 24hr urinary free cortisol (nmol/24h) | 502 | < 350 |
| Plasma ACTH at 0900h (ng/L) | 263 | 9-52 |

*POINTS:*

1. Ectopic ACTH production from carcinoma of the bronchus is a recognised cause of Cushing's syndrome. The excess corticosteroid production causes hypokalaemia and hyperglycaemia. Hypercortisolaemia results in increased hepatic gluconeogenesis and hepatic glucose output as well as stimulating lipolysis and protein catabolism. Glucose intolerance is found in 80-90% of cases of Cushing's syndrome and frank diabetes in 15-20 %.

2. Palmar pigmentation, identical to that of Addison's disease, results from the excessive circulating ACTH.

3. Although initial LFTs were normal, this does not exclude the possibility of liver secondaries.

4. Insulin should be used to treat the diabetes but the prognosis is poor.

AN UNUSUAL PRESENTATION OF DIABETES IN A YOUNG GIRL

A 15 year old girl attended her family doctor complaining of tiredness. Her mother and grandmother were known to have diabetes and her 24-year-old sister had recently been found to have gestational diabetes.

Because of this family history the family doctor arranged for her to have a glucose tolerance test. The results showed a fasting plasma glucose of 7.2 mmol/L and a 2-hour plasma glucose of 13.1 mmol/L. She was referred to the local hospital diabetes clinic. When seen there the family history was noted. She weighed 55.5 kg and her BMI was 23 kg/m$^2$. Physical examination was unremarkable.

Given the family history and the mild nature of the biochemical abnormality it was suggested that she might have MODY (maturity onset diabetes of the young) and blood was sent for genetic analysis. This confirmed a mutation of the glucokinase gene.

*POINTS:*

1. MODY should be suspected when autosomal dominant inheritance is inferred. Diabetes of similar phenotype should be present in at least two generations and preferably three. Diagnosis before the age of 25 should have been made in one first degree relative and preferably two.

2. It is rarely appropriate to call diabetes 'mild' and even in the MODY syndrome, some mutations result in diabetes that requires insulin treatment and that leads to complications. In glucokinase mutations, the biochemical disorder tends to be mild, treatment is with diet or a small dose of an insulin secretagogue and significant complications are uncommon.

3. Recognition of this type of diabetes is important. The family can be reassured of the nature of this type of diabetes. Confirmation of the genetic abnormality can reassure the clinician that this does not represent an unusual presentation of type 1 diabetes in a young person.

# Chapter 2

# The pathophysiology of diabetes

## THE HISTOLOGY OF THE PANCREAS IN DIABETES

The importance of the pancreas in diabetes became apparent when it was found that diabetes could be produced experimentally by removing it. This led to concentrated study on the islets of Langerhans. For many years, however, interpretation of the histology of the pancreas in diabetic patients was hampered by diabetes being considered as one disease. It should not be forgotten that as little as 30 years ago, type 2 diabetes, or maturity-onset diabetes as it was then called, was simply regarded as a milder form of type 1 diabetes, then known as juvenile-onset diabetes. Appreciation of the clear distinction in both aetiology and pathogenesis between the two major types of diabetes has come about relatively recently.

*Hyaline change* was first described about one hundred years ago. Hyaline material is found in relation to the capillaries, usually between the lumina of the sinusoids and the β cells, and can sometimes obliterate the whole islet. The involvement of islets is patchy, some remaining normal when others are severely involved. Hyaline possesses the ultrastructural features of amyloid on electron micrographs and is distinct from the basement membrane thickening of microangiopathy. Islet amyloid is much more common in elderly patients with diabetes than in the young and is found in 50-90% of diabetic patients over the age of 40. The precursor of amyloid has been identified and termed diabetes-associated-peptide or islet amyloid polypeptide. The peptide has similarities to calcitonin gene-related peptide and, to a lesser extent, the A chain of insulin.

*Fibrosis* entails the formation of a fibrous capsule round the islet with infiltration of fibroblasts. Although seen in children, it is more often found in older subjects, particularly in association with chronic pancreatitis.

*Hydropic change* consists of a foamy and, later, vacuolated appearance of the β cells. In experimental diabetes, it is the earliest sign of injury to the β cells and is reversible if the provocative agent is removed. In man, its significance is unclear. In many, if not all patients, it has been shown to be due to infiltration with glycogen, as occurs in many organs in diabetes. Therefore, it may not necessarily reflect a specific pancreatic pathological change.

*Lymphocytic infiltration* is a particular feature of the pancreas of young patients with diabetes of acute onset. The islets are reduced in size and cellularity, and those remaining are generally arranged in narrow cords. Beta cells are more severely involved than α cells. The infiltration is of variable degree and may be accompanied by moderate fibrosis. The inflammatory response that this signals has been termed insulitis. It is thought to represent a response to viral infection or an immunological attack.

*Small islets with few β cells* have been observed in large numbers of both type 1 and type 2 diabetic patients, although the reduction is most marked in younger type 1 patients. This finding would appear to correlate with chemical analysis of the diabetic pancreas and, specifically, estimation of the amount of insulin in the pancreas. There is very little insulin within pancreases from type 1 diabetic patients whereas those from patients with type 2 diabetes contain about half of the normal amount.

*Arterial or arteriolar narrowing* in the blood supply to the islets is a common finding in diabetic patients, particularly the elderly, although its significance is uncertain.

In summary, the pancreas is often normal in size in type 1 diabetes at diagnosis but microscopy reveals lymphocytic infiltration of the islets, so-called insulitis. This infiltration does not occur in a uniform way: some islets may show β cell loss and fibrosis while others may be apparently normal. In long-standing type 1 diabetes, islets of Langerhans are small, resulting from an almost total absence of β cells with a degree of fibrosis. Other secretory cells, e.g. α, δ and pancreatic polypeptide secreting cells, are present in normal numbers.

In type 2 diabetes there is a reduction in β cell mass to about 50% of normal although this is not a constant finding and there is considerable overlap with the non-diabetic pancreas. The most consistent finding is amyloid deposition, considered the commonest and most typical lesion of the pancreas in type 2 diabetes. Fibrosis also occurs frequently although the precise stimulus to the fibrosis remains unclear.

## THE PATHOGENESIS OF TYPE 1 DIABETES

### INSULIN
The human insulin gene is located on the short arm of chromosome 11. It is 1355 base pairs long made up of 2 introns and 3 exons (coding regions). There is some species-specific allelic variation but in the main there is a remarkable similarity throughout nature. In the non-coding regions, particularly the 5'-flanking region, there is considerable within-species variation.

**The structure of insulin**

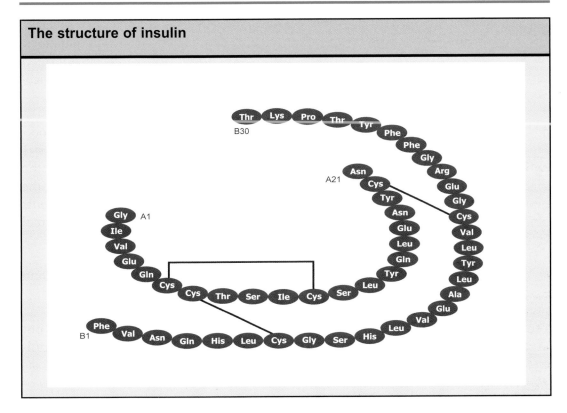

**Figure 2.1 Insulin comprises two polypeptide chains linked by two disulphide bridges**

There is no doubt that in biochemical terms, insulin deficiency is the crucial factor in the pathogenesis of type 1 diabetes. Insulin is synthesised in the β cells of the islets of Langerhans of the pancreas via a number of precursors. The first to be identified was proinsulin, the structure of which explained the two chain structure of insulin. The A and B chains of the insulin molecule are joined by disulphide bridges. In proinsulin, the ends of the A and B chains are linked by a polypeptide known as connecting peptide (or C-peptide); thus proinsulin is a single polypeptide chain. In mature secretory granules, connecting peptide is removed, releasing equimolar quantities of insulin and C-peptide into the circulation. Proinsulin itself is derived from a precursor, preproinsulin, which has an additional 24 residue peptide chain.

METABOLIC EFFECTS OF INSULIN

*HEPATIC EFFECTS OF INSULIN*
The liver has a crucial role in regulating blood glucose concentration. In the fasting state, circulating glucose concentration is maintained predominantly by release of

glucose from the liver. This is particularly important for brain and a number of other tissues for which glucose is the major metabolic fuel, and in which uptake of glucose is concentration dependent rather than insulin dependent. Hepatic glucose output involves both the release of stored carbohydrate, glycogenolysis, and synthesis of the 6-carbon compound glucose from 3-carbon precursors, gluconeogenesis.

*Glycogen synthesis* is the conversion of glucose to the polymeric form for storage. Entry of glucose into the liver is independent of insulin. The first step in intracellular metabolism is the conversion of glucose to glucose 6-phosphate by the enzyme glucokinase. Through glucose 6-phosphate, a small amount of glucose enters hepatic glycolysis but the majority is stored as glycogen. The first step is the conversion of glucose 6-phosphate to glucose 1-phosphate, from which glycogen synthesis is regulated by glycogen synthase. The activation of this enzyme is through a dephosphorylation/phosphorylation cycle regulated by a cyclic AMP dependent protein kinase. Glycogen synthesis and glycogen breakdown are reciprocally linked, with glycogenolysis being regulated by phosphorylase. Phosphorylase is regulated by the same cyclic AMP dependent protein kinase. This enzyme is activated and deactivated through a phosphorylation/dephosphorylation cascade. The active form of phosphorylase is the phosphorylated form, while for glycogen synthase it is the dephosphorylated form.

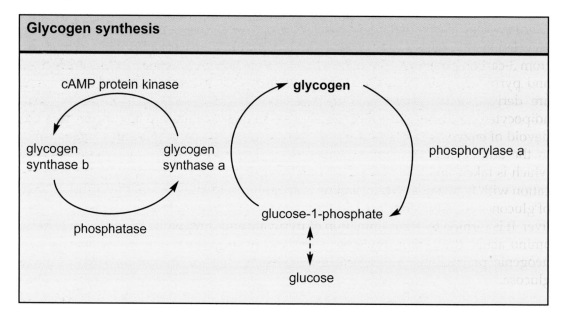

**Glycogen synthesis**

Figure 2.2 Glycogen is synthesized from glucose 1-phosphate in reactions catalyzed by glycogen synthase a, an enzyme that is activated by dephosphorylation of glycogen synthase b (inactive)

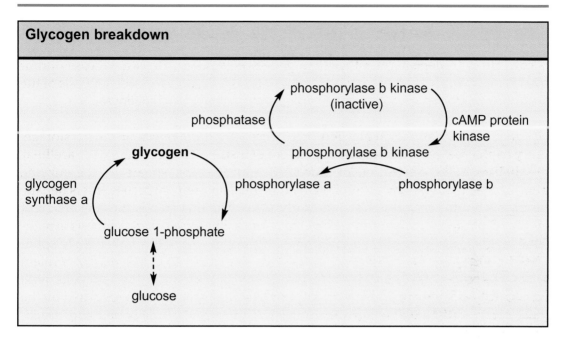

**Figure 2.3 Glycogenolysis is catalyzed principally by phosphorylase a, an enzyme that is activated by phosphorylation of phosphorylase b (inactive)**

*Gluconeogenesis* is the hepatic pathway by which substrates released peripherally are recycled to glucose. Gluconeogenesis involves the synthesis of a 6-carbon compound from 3-carbon skeletons. The main substrates for hepatic gluconeogenesis are lactate and pyruvate, amino acids, especially alanine, and glycerol. Lactate and pyruvate are derived from partial oxidative metabolism in tissues such as muscle and adipocytes, and from anaerobic metabolism in cells such as red blood cells that are devoid of enzymes of the tricarboxylic acid cycle. Glycerol comes from triglycerides in the adipocytes. The carbon skeleton of glycerol also originates from glucose, which is taken up by the fat cells and converted to α-glycerophosphate for esterification with fatty acids. While alanine is an amino acid in its own right, in the context of gluconeogenesis it functions as a transporter of nitrogen from the periphery to the liver. It is formed by transamination of pyruvate and thus, while the nitrogen is from amino acids, the carbon skeleton is derived from glucose. Thus the major gluconeogenic precursors all have carbon skeletons that are derived ultimately from glucose.

Gluconeogenesis is regulated in several ways, including alteration in substrate supply to the liver, alteration in hepatic extraction of substrate from the blood and intrahepatic modulation. All of these steps are targets for hormonal action and allow direct and indirect regulation of gluconeogenesis by insulin.

**Hepatic glucose production**

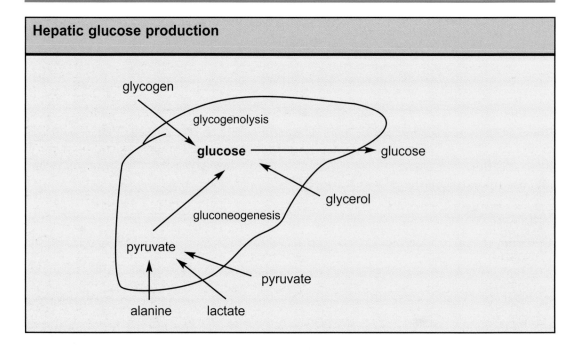

**Figure 2.4 Gluconeogenesis can occur from pyruvate, from lactate and alanine via pyruvate, and from glycerol via α-glycerophosphate**

*Lipogenesis,* or fat synthesis, is also a function of the liver. Dietary fat, plasma non-esterified fatty acids and *de novo* synthesis of fatty acids from glucose contribute to hepatic triglyceride synthesis and subsequent release. Fatty acid synthesis within the liver is from acetyl CoA derived from carbohydrate sources. Acetyl CoA is carboxylated to form malonyl CoA by the enzyme acetyl CoA carboxylase. Malonyl CoA undergoes repeated addition of acetyl CoA units until the required chain length is reached. In man, the major product is palmitoyl CoA. Other fatty acids are formed by saturation, desaturation, and hydroxyl addition.

Acetyl CoA carboxylase appears to be the main site of regulation. Low insulin concentrations, as are found in starvation or alloxan-induced diabetes in animals, reduce fatty acid biosynthesis; this can be reversed by refeeding or insulin.

*PERIPHERAL EFFECTS OF INSULIN*

*Peripheral glucose uptake and metabolism*
The major proportion of glucose uptake by muscle and adipose tissue is insulin dependent. Muscle accounts for 85% of total body glucose uptake and adipose tissue accounts for a further 10%. Even in these tissues, however, some glucose uptake is mediated by the prevailing glucose concentration but in other tissues, namely liver,

brain and nerve (including the retina), renal medulla and erythrocytes, glucose uptake is entirely independent of insulin.

Glucose uptake into tissues is mediated by a family of membrane proteins called glucose transporters, which display some tissue specificity. For example GLUT 2 is the major glucose transporter of liver, kidney and β cell, while GLUT 4 is the major transporter of skeletal and cardiac muscle and of adipose tissue. Although there is evidence for an effect of insulin upon the translocation of GLUT 4 from an intracellular location to the plasma membrane, the precise site of insulin regulation of glucose uptake remains unclear.

| Glucose transporters | |
| --- | --- |
| **Transporter** | **Tissue distribution** |
| GLUT 1 | brain, erythrocytes, kidney, fetal tissue |
| GLUT 2 | liver, kidney, pancreatic β cells |
| GLUT 3 | fetal muscle |
| GLUT 4 | skeletal and cardiac muscle, adipose tissue |
| GLUT 5 | small intestine |

**Figure 2.5  Glucose transporters**

A key step in glucose oxidation lies at the transition from anaerobic glycolysis in the cytosol to aerobic metabolism in the tricarboxylic acid cycle in mitochondria. The conversion of pyruvate to acetyl CoA by pyruvate dehydrogenase is irreversible, and therefore represents a potential loss of carbohydrate stores. The benefits, however, are that other metabolic pathways, such as fatty acid and cholesterol synthesis are opened up, and a supply of substrate for copious energy production is obtained. Pyruvate dehydrogenase is an enzyme complex regulated by phosphorylation/ dephosphorylation. The balance between the phosphorylated enzyme (inactive) and dephosphorylated enzyme (active) is regulated through kinase and phosphatase enzymes. Regulation of the kinase is by ratios of acetyl CoA:CoA, NADH:NAD$^+$, and ATP:ADP, an increase in any of these ratios activating the kinase and therefore inactivating pyruvate dehydrogenase. Insulin increases the proportion of active to inactive pyruvate dehydrogenase. It is not entirely clear whether, *in vivo*, this is a direct effect or is mediated through changes in the concentrations of metabolites, for example, fatty acids and ketone bodies.

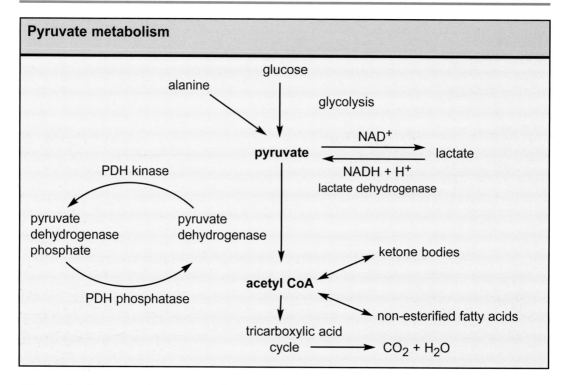

**Pyruvate metabolism**

Figure 2.6 Pyruvate is converted to acetyl CoA in a reaction catalyzed by pyruvate dehydrogenase; this enzyme is active when dephosphorylated and inactive when phosphorylated

*Protein metabolism*
Protein synthesis from amino acids involves cellular uptake, activation and polymerisation, providing numerous sites for regulation. Insulin deficiency results in reduced protein synthesis, which can be corrected by insulin administration. Increasing circulating concentrations of amino acids by feeding also stimulates protein synthesis, although this effect is somewhat offset by the effect of insulin in lowering circulating concentrations of amino acids. Insulin appears also to inhibit proteolysis.

*Fat metabolism*
The storage fat of adipose tissue is triglyceride. Triglyceride is synthesised within adipocytes from fatty acids and α-glycerophosphate. At the endothelial surface, triglyceride, which originates in the liver, is degraded by lipoprotein lipase, releasing fatty acids that pass into the cell. Here they are reesterified with α-glycerophosphate to form triglyceride. The glycerophosphate is derived from glucose, not glycerol, since human adipocytes do not contain the enzyme α-glycerokinase. The activity of lipoprotein lipase and glucose uptake into the fat cell are both increased by insulin.

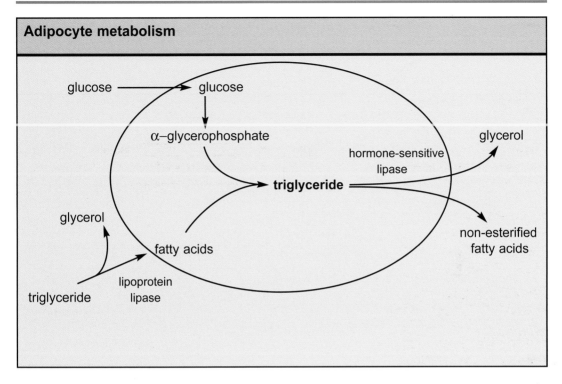

**Adipocyte metabolism**

**Figure 2.7 Triglycerides in chylomicrons and very low density lipoproteins are hydrolysed by lipoprotein lipase (which is activated by insulin). The non-esterified fatty acids are reesterified to triglyceride for storage. Hydrolysis of this triglyceride by hormone-sensitive lipase (inhibited by insulin) releases non-esterified fatty acids and glycerol into the bloodstream.**

Triglyceride is broken down into fatty acids and glycerol in the process known as lipolysis. The lack of α-glycerokinase means that glycerol cannot be used in reesterification and it is therefore released. Its ultimate fate is to be taken up by the liver for gluconeogenesis. Some of the fatty acids generated in this way are used in reesterification and the remainder is released into the circulation. Breakdown of triglyceride is controlled by hormone-sensitive lipase, which is extremely sensitive to inhibition by insulin.

Non-esterified fatty acids are taken up by the liver down a concentration gradient. Metabolism is by intramitochondrial β-oxidation. Mitochondrial uptake requires creation of the fatty acyl CoA derivative, which is then linked to carnitine by carnitine acyl transferase I (CAT 1) on the outer mitochondrial membrane. Carnitine acyl transferase II (CAT II), on the inner mitochondrial membrane, splits off carnitine, leaving fatty acyl CoA inside the mitochondrion.

In the liver, fatty acids may undergo complete β-oxidation to acetyl CoA and thence via the tricarboxylic acid cycle to carbon dioxide and water; be partially oxidised to acetyl CoA followed by condensation to acetoacetyl CoA and thence ketone bodies, or be reesterified with subsequent release of very low density lipoprotein (VLDL).

There is an intimate relationship between ketogenesis and fatty acid synthesis. Ketogenesis is regulated through malonyl CoA, the first committed intermediate of fatty acid synthesis. When there is a good supply of substrate for fatty acid synthesis, that is in the fed state, the high concentration of malonyl CoA inhibits ketogenesis. In the fasting state, low concentrations allow ketone body synthesis. Glucagon, which increases ketogenesis, lowers malonyl CoA concentration. The role of insulin in regulating ketogenesis is unclear and it may be that it is the insulin/glucagon ratio in portal blood that is important.

## CHANGES IN TYPE 1 DIABETES
In insulin deficiency, blood glucose concentrations are raised owing to overproduction by the liver and underutilisation by the periphery. With the high circulating glucose concentration, non-insulin mediated glucose uptake is enhanced in both metabolically active tissues. Partial oxidation of glucose in these tissues leads to enhanced release of lactate and pyruvate, which further drive gluconeogenesis to produce glucose.

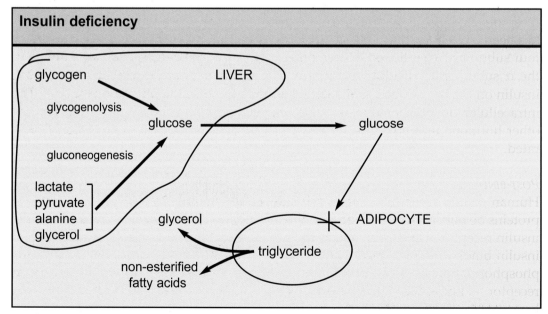

Figure 2.8 **Insulin deficiency results in increased glycogenolysis and gluconeogenesis in the liver; in adipocytes, lipolysis is increased and glucose uptake is decreased**

With regard to protein metabolism, insulin deficiency causes enhanced proteolysis and decreased synthesis, leading to negative nitrogen balance.

Fat metabolism is also affected, with decreased storage of fat and increased break-down, resulting in high plasma non-esterified fatty acid concentrations. Within the liver, the hormonal milieu favours ketone body synthesis.

The differential sensitivity of metabolic processes to insulin is often under-appreci-ated. Lipolysis is exquisitely sensitive to inhibition by insulin, circulating concentra-tions of 10 mU/L (little higher than fasting concentrations in normal subjects) having a demonstrable effect, while stimulation of glucose uptake into muscle and adipose tissue requires concentrations 5-10 times greater. Thus raised fatty acid concentrations and the presence of ketone bodies are a sign of marked insulin defi-ciency.

## PATHOGENESIS OF TYPE 2 DIABETES

### INSULIN RESISTANCE

#### INSULIN RECEPTORS
The first step in the action of insulin is binding to a specific receptor. This is followed by initation and amplification of the signal leading to the metabolic action. Insulin receptors are large glycoprotein components of tissue plasma membranes. The gene has been cloned and is localised to chromosome 19. An insulin receptor consists of four subunits; two α linked to each other by disulphide bridges, and two β linked to the α subunits by disulphide bridges. The α subunits are extracellular and bind insulin on the cell surface, while the β subunits traverse the plasma membrane. The intracellular domain includes a tyrosine-specific protein kinase. In common with other hormone receptors, insulin receptors are specific and can be reversibly satu-rated.

#### POST-BINDING EVENTS
Human insulin receptors express tyrosine kinase activity. Not only can exogenous proteins be phosphorylated but autophosphorylation of tyrosine residues within the insulin receptor also occurs, owing to immediate activation of tyrosine kinase when insulin binds to the receptor. Thus it appears that autophosphorylation or perhaps phosphorylation of other proteins in response to insulin binding to the insulin receptor is crucial for signal transmission. A number of other intracellular proteins have been identified that may be implicated. One of these is insulin receptor substrate 1 (IRS-1), and it is possible that phosphorylation of tyrosine residues on this, or similar proteins, by the insulin receptor tyrosine kinase, may be the initiator of intracellular insulin action.

*HYPERINSULINAEMIA*

Hyperinsulinism is found in obese people with normal glucose tolerance, suggesting that they have some degree of resistance to insulin.

In type 2 diabetic patients, however, and in patients with impaired glucose tolerance, modern immunoradiometric assays have shown elevated fasting plasma concentrations of proinsulin and split products of proinsulin. However, it has been harder to confirm raised insulin concentrations in these patients. Fortunately, a variety of other techniques have been used to demonstrate that insulin resistance is present in patients with type 2 diabetes.

## METHODS OF STUDYING INSULIN RESISTANCE

Insulin action can be studied by measurement of fasting glucose and insulin concentrations, stimulatory tests such as the oral glucose tolerance test and euglycaemic or hyperglycaemic clamping.

Glucose clamping is perhaps the favoured technique because it gives a clear numerical value and allows construction of dose-response curves. An infusion of glucose is used to maintain the starting blood glucose during infusions of insulin designed to produce logarithmically increasing circulating insulin concentrations of, say, 100, 1,000 and 10,000 mU/L. The combination of insulin infusion to a circulating concentration of 100 mU/L with glucose infusion effectively blocks hepatic glucose output. Under these steady-state conditions, the amount of glucose infused to maintain blood glucose concentration must equal the amount that is being taken up by peripheral tissues, thus giving an indirect measure of glucose disposal. Clearly, the lower the amount of glucose uptake by the tissues, the greater is the insulin resistance.

In interpreting the results obtained using this technique, it is assumed that hepatic glucose production is effectively blocked at insulin concentrations that are similar in normal and insulin resistant subjects. This may not be valid. Thus isotopic methods are employed to measure glucose turnover and obtain results from which to derive measures of endogenous glucose output and peripheral glucose uptake.

## INSULIN SECRETION IN TYPE 2 DIABETES

Interpretation of some studies of hyperinsulinaemia is difficult. Matching diabetic patients and controls for body weight has not always been given sufficient attention. It is clear that if oral glucose tolerance tests are performed in obese type 2 diabetic patients and the results compared with those from non-diabetic lean controls, the obese diabetic patients will have higher blood glucose and plasma insulin concentration than the lean non-diabetic patients, leading to the conclusion that they are insulin resistant. If matched with appropriate obese non-diabetic controls, however, insulin responses in the diabetic patients are reduced, leading to the conclusion that there is also an element of insulin deficiency.

When intravenous glucose is used as a stimulus to insulin secretion, the response in normal subjects is biphasic. It is suggested that the first phase of insulin release is from a readily releasable pool of synthesised insulin and that second phase insulin release is the slower release of newly synthesised insulin. In type 2 diabetes, first phase insulin secretion is markedly diminished or lost. Inadequate first phase insulin release results in hyperglycaemia, and thus a greater stimulus to second phase secretion, and hence second phase secretion is exaggerated. This situation persists until the more severely hyperglycaemic stage of the disease is reached, when second phase response also becomes impaired.

Thus it is now widely accepted that both insulin resistance and diminished insulin secretion contribute to the pathogenesis of type 2 diabetes, although the molecular basis of neither mechanism is fully understood.

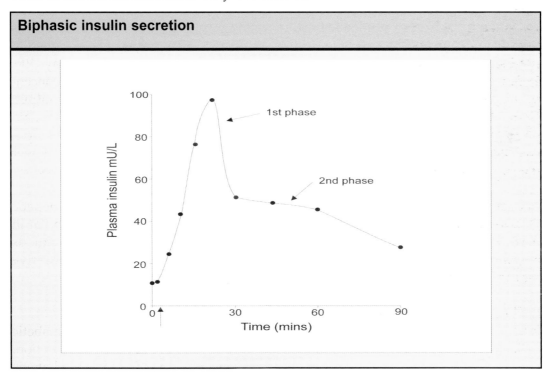

**Figure 2.9 Insulin secretion following a bolus intravenous injection of glucose, showing the normal biphasic response**

## FURTHER READING

Bell GI, Swain WF, Pictet RL *et al*. Sequence of the human insulin gene. Nature 1980; **284:** 26-32.

De Fronzo RA, Tobin JD, Andres R. Glucose clamp technique: a method for quantifying insulin secretion and resistance. Am J Physiol 1979; **237:** 214-23.

Himsworth HP. Diabetes mellitus; its differentiation into insulin sensitive and insulin-insensitive types. Lancet 1936; **I:** 127-30.

Owerbach D, Bell GI, Rutter WJ *et al*. The insulin gene is located on the short arm of chromosome 11 in humans. Diabetes 1981; **30:** 267-70.

Porte D, Pupo AA. Insulin responses to glucose: evidence for a two pool system in man. J Clin Invest 1969; **48:** 2309-19.

Randle PJ, Garland PB, Hales CN, Newsholme EA. The glucose fatty-acid cycle. Its role in insulin sensitivity and the metabolic disturbances of diabetes. Lancet 1963; **I:** 785-9.

Reaven GM. Role of insulin resistance in human disease. Diabetes 1988; **37:** 1595-607.

Ullrich A, Bell JR, Chen EY *et al*. Human insulin receptor and its relationship to the tyrosine kinase family of oncogenes. Nature 1985; **313:** 756-61.

Westermark P, Wernstedt C, Wilander E *et al*. Amyloid fibrils in human insulinoma and islets of Langerhans of the diabetic cat are derived from neuropeptide-like protein also present in normal cells. Proc Nat Acad Sci USA 1987; **84:** 3881-5.

# CLINICAL CASES

## PRESENTATION OF ?TYPE 1 DIABETES

A 37 year old woman presented with a four week history of thirst and polyuria. She had lost 7.5 kg in weight over the preceding six weeks. On examination she looked well.

A random plasma glucose measurement was 19.6 mmol/L. Her urine contained glucose +++ but no ketones.

The only significant finding on examination was her weight (109.2 kg), which, for her height of 165 cms, gave her a BMI of 39.8 kg/m$^2$.

*POINTS:*

1. After confirmation of the diagnosis the next important issue is classification, that is, what type of diabetes does this patient have? A young person with newly diagnosed diabetes, a short history of acute symptoms and weight loss, almost certainly has type 1 diabetes, whereas an older person who is asymptomatic, obese and has not lost weight is likely to have type 2 diabetes.

2. Weight loss is an important pointer to the type of diabetes. Relatively low circulating concentrations of insulin inhibit fat breakdown. If fat is being broken down, the implication is that, despite a circulating glucose of, say, 20 mmol/L, the amount of insulin being secreted is insufficient to inhibit the process. Therefore, the patient is likely to have type 1 diabetes.

3. Difficulties arise when the presentation is slightly unusual and particularly when weight loss is a significant finding yet the patient is still obese.

4. Measurement of circulating insulin or C-peptide is rarely useful since there are major difficulties in interpreting concentrations in relation to the raised circulating glucose. If it is important to be sure of the type of diabetes then measurement of islet cell antibodies or GAD antibodies is appropriate.

5. In the majority of patients who present in this way the correct approach to treatment would be insulin with a note to review the situation in 3-6 months.

PRESENTATION OF ?TYPE 2 DIABETES

A 54 year old man was admitted to the coronary care unit following a myocardial infarction, which was confirmed on ECG and CK measurement. A reagent stick measurement of blood glucose was 10.1 mmol/L and blood was sent to the laboratory for measurement of glucose and $HbA_{1c}$. His plasma glucose 8 h after the onset of pain was 14.3 mmol/L and his $HbA_{1c}$ was 6.9% (reference range < 6.0%). His urine was tested and found to contain ++ of ketones.

He was commenced on treatment with an insulin and glucose infusion for 72 hours. Following this, he was transferred to four times daily insulin. His recovery was uneventful and he was discharged on this treatment.

He was seen in the diabetes clinic three months later when he was well. His plasma glucose concentration in the clinic was 6.2 mmol/L and $HbA_{1c}$ 5.6%. He had not had any hypoglycaemic events. His insulin treatment was continued.

*POINTS:*

1. Screening for diabetes on a coronary care unit will reveal a number of patients not previously known to have diabetes.

2. The catabolic response to a myocardial infarction includes catecholamine release which, in addition to central effects upon the liver and peripheral effects upon muscle and fat tissue, also inhibits insulin secretion. When marked, this can lead to ketonuria. Upon recovery and decrease in circulating catecholamines to normal, sufficient insulin secretion may return to maintain normal or near normal plasma glucose concentrations. This highly catabolic situation is one of the very few occasions when ketonuria does not imply insulin dependence (i.e. type 1 diabetes).

3. Given the clinical presentation and the subsequent progress of this patient it is more likely that he has type 2 diabetes. There is good evidence, however that treatment of diabetes with insulin following a myocardial infarction leads to an improvement in outcome.

# Chapter 3

# The diagnosis of diabetes

A diagnosis of diabetes mellitus has serious consequences for an individual's future lifestyle. It means a lifetime of dietary restriction and probable medication, with the knowledge that the long-term complications of the disease may lead to blindness or limb amputation, and that there is an increased likelihood of coronary vascular disease. The types of activities and employment a person with diabetes can take up are restricted and life assurance is likely to be more difficult to obtain, with higher premiums to pay. Accurate diagnosis is therefore essential.

## GLUCOSE MEASUREMENT

The diagnosis of diabetes mellitus is made on the basis of plasma (or blood) glucose measurements. Glucose may be measured on whole blood or plasma specimens and both venous and capillary samples can be used. The preferred specimen is venous plasma, which should be harvested from blood collected into a suitable anticoagulant containing an antiglycolytic agent (usually sodium fluoride). Serum should not be used because glucose in the specimen will be metabolised during any delay prior to centrifugation.

In the laboratory, methods for glucose measurement must be subject to rigid internal quality control procedures and external quality assessment. The World Health Organisation (WHO) recommends that glucose measurements used for diagnostic purposes are carried out in an accredited laboratory, using a specific enzymatic method. Reagent strips and glucose meters should not be used for diagnosis. However, such devices have a major part to play in monitoring glycaemic control in people with established diabetes, and may have a role in initial screening.

There are significant differences between glucose concentrations measured in equivalent whole blood and plasma samples, and between capillary and venous blood; it is essential that this is taken into account when considering a diagnosis of diabetes mellitus. The diagnostic criteria issued by the World Health Organization (*see Figure 3.1*) are based on glucose concentrations and clearly differentiate between the critical values for the different types of specimen. *All glucose concentrations quoted in the text of this chapter relate to results obtained on plasma harvested from venous blood.*

| WHO diagnostic criteria for diabetes | | | | |
|---|---|---|---|---|
| | Glucose concentration (mmol/L) | | | |
| | Whole blood | | Plasma | |
| | Venous | Capillary | Venous | Capillary |
| **Normal** | | | | |
| Fasting | < 5.6 | < 5.6 | < 6.1 | < 6.1 |
| 2h post glucose load* | < 6.7 | < 7.8 | < 7.8 | < 8.9 |
| **Diabetes Mellitus** | | | | |
| Fasting | ≥ 6.1 | ≥ 6.1 | ≥ 7.0 | ≥ 7.0 |
| *and/or* 2h post glucose load | ≥ 10.0 | ≥ 11.1 | ≥ 11.1 | ≥ 12.2 |
| **Impaired glucose tolerance (IGT)** | | | | |
| Fasting | < 6.1 | < 6.1 | < 7.0 | < 7.0 |
| *and/or* 2h post glucose load | ≥ 6.7 & <10.0 | ≥ 7.8 & < 11.1 | ≥ 7.8 & < 11.1 | ≥ 8.9 & < 12.2 |
| **Impaired fasting glycaemia (IFG)** | | | | |
| Fasting | ≥ 5.6 & < 6.1 | ≥ 5.6 & < 6.1 | ≥ 6.1 & < 7.0 | ≥ 6.1 & < 7.0 |
| *and* 2h post glucose load | < 6.7 | < 7.8 | < 7.8 | < 8.9 |

\* glucose load: 75g anhydrous glucose or equivalent

**Figure 3.1 World Health Organisation diagnostic criteria for diabetes mellitus and the states of impaired glucose regulation**

OTHER BIOCHEMICAL PARAMETERS

Alternative biochemical measurements for the diagnosis of diabetes have been suggested, most notably glycated haemoglobin ($HbA_{1c}$). At present, however, the use of glycated haemoglobin is not recommended for diagnosis. Lack of standardisation of $HbA_{1c}$ assays (*see Chapter 6*), and the method dependent contribution of haemoglobin variants to results, are particular problems. However, the role of $HbA_{1c}$ measurements in the diagnosis of DM is likely to be reconsidered in the future, as technological developments lead to simple, more robust analytical systems that can be made more widely available.

PLASMA GLUCOSE AND DIAGNOSIS

In many cases, the diagnosis of diabetes is obvious clinically, and plasma glucose measurement is required only for confirmation. However, for patients who present with vague symptoms, or when there is only a strong clinical suspicion, perhaps linked to other factors such as ethnicity or a positive family history, proper use of glucose measurements can establish or eliminate the diagnosis. In addition, because of the prevalence of the disease, many clinicians include a random blood glucose measurement in the investigations they request in connection with routine referrals.

The spectrum of presenting features in DM is broad. Some patients present with severe, characteristic symptoms of the disease, such as weight loss, thirst and polyuria and, occasionally, most frequently in children, with diabetic ketoacidosis. Others present at an earlier stage of the disease process with few, if any, symptoms, but significant hyperglycaemia.

In patients with characteristic symptoms of diabetes, a single random glucose value above the defined level establishes the diagnosis. However, it should be remembered that metabolic stress, which occurs following trauma, in severe infection and in acute illness, can be associated with hyperglycaemia, and a diagnosis of DM should *not* be made under these circumstances. For individuals presenting with minor symptoms, biochemical confirmation of the diagnosis is essential, by measurement of fasting or random, plasma or blood glucose concentration in the first instance and, if there is still doubt, by challenging the ability of the individual to handle a glucose load, using the oral glucose tolerance test (OGTT). Diabetes mellitus should *never* be diagnosed on a single blood glucose concentration in patients without characteristic symptoms.

## DIAGNOSTIC CRITERIA
The recommended diagnostic criteria for DM have been modified over the years. The high morbidity and mortality associated with poorly controlled DM makes it imperative to diagnose the condition at an early stage and to identify those who do not have DM *per se* but are at increased likelihood of developing the disease or the long term macrovascular complications associated with it.

Since recommendations were first published, fasting, random and glucose concentrations following administration of a glucose load have all been included in the diagnostic criteria for the biochemical diagnosis of DM. The first of these to be internationally recognised came from reports of the WHO Expert Committee and were subsequently updated by the WHO Study Group on Diabetes Mellitus. In the USA, the National Diabetes Data Group (NDDG) and the American Diabetes Association (ADA) have published several reports recommending diagnostic criteria. Some, but not all of these, have been incorporated into the current WHO criteria.

The key discriminative glucose concentrations specified in the 1985 WHO report were:

- a random glucose concentration less than 5.6 mmol/L makes DM unlikely

- a random glucose greater than 11.0 mmol/L establishes the diagnosis.

The scientific basis for the selection of these figures is doubtful: 5.5 mmol/L and 11.1 mmol/L simply equate to 100 mg/dL and 200 mg/dL, the units still used in the USA.

In addition, for glucose concentrations in response to an oral glucose load equivalent to 75 g glucose:

- a fasting glucose concentration greater than 7.8 mmol/L and/or a two hour glucose concentration greater than 11.0 mmol/L establish the diagnosis

- a fasting glucose less than 7.8 mmol/L and a two hour glucose greater than 7.8 mmol/L but less than 11.1 mmol/L, establish a diagnosis of impaired glucose tolerance (IGT).

The diagnostic criteria currently in use in the UK are those published by the WHO in 1999 and endorsed by Diabetes UK (formerly the British Diabetic Association) the following year. The criteria refine those in the previous WHO reports. In the new recommendations, there are several important changes:

- the fasting glucose concentration for the diagnosis of DM is lowered from 7.8 mmol/L to 7.0 mmol/L

- the definition of a new diagnostic category, impaired fasting glycaemia (IFG), in which the fasting glucose concentration is greater than 6.0 mmol/L and less than 7.0 mmol/L

- a statement that glycated haemoglobin measurement should not be used to diagnose DM

- a statement that the glucose load administered in an oral glucose tolerance test (OGTT) should be the equivalent of 75 g *anhydrous* glucose and that it is necessary to collect only fasting and two hour specimens for glucose measurement to permit diagnosis.

## THE ORAL GLUCOSE TOLERANCE TEST

The gold standard investigation for the diagnosis of DM is the OGTT, and the WHO recommends that this should be performed when random glucose values fall in the range where the diagnosis is classified as 'uncertain'. The minimum requirements of the OGTT, as defined by the WHO are:

• unrestricted diet for three days prior to test, with a daily intake of at least 150 g of carbohydrate and normal physical activity

• 8-14 hour overnight fast

• no smoking, eating, drinking or exercise during the test

• fasting blood specimen for glucose measurement

• 75 g anhydrous glucose (or equivalent) load, in 250-300 mL water, to be taken over a five minute period

• blood specimen two hours after glucose ingestion for glucose measurement.

The blood specimens should be analysed as soon as possible. If delays in measurement are anticipated, plasma harvested from the centrifuged blood specimens should be frozen until analysis.

For children, the glucose load should be the equivalent of 1.75 g glucose per kg body weight, up to a maximum total load of 75 g.

In the UK, it is usual to administer proprietary preparations, containing glucose polymers, as the carbohydrate load. Many of these are flavoured to make them more palatable and they may cause less nausea than solutions made by dissolving glucose in water. Care must always be taken to ensure that the correct volume is given to achieve the equivalent of a total load of 75 g anhydrous glucose.

Interpretation of glucose values obtained during the OGTT is shown in Figure 3.1; a schematic representation showing how the diagnosis of DM and associated states of impaired glucose handling is shown in Figure 3.2.

**Diagnostic algorithm for the diagnosis of diabetes mellitus**

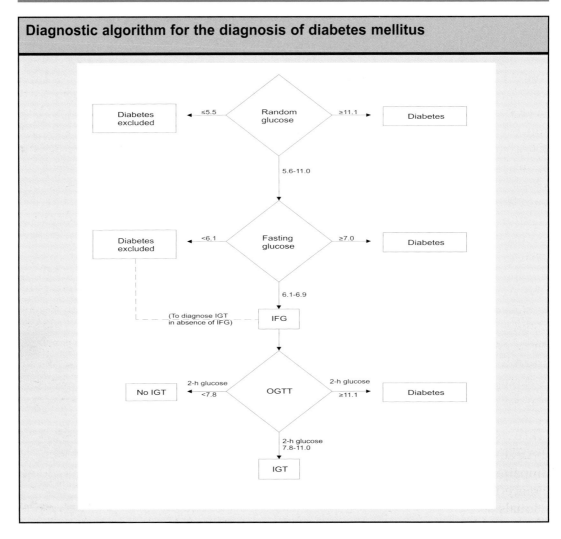

**Figure 3.2 Diagnostic algorithm for the diagnosis of diabetes mellitus (Lamb EJ, Day AP. Reproduced with permission from Annals of Clinical Biochemistry)**

## WHY MODIFY THE CRITERIA?

It is now well recognised that a fasting glucose concentration above 7.8 mmol/L does not predict all individuals who have a two hour glucose concentration greater than 11.0 mmol/L in an OGTT. Using that cut-off, the diagnosis of DM will be missed in a significant number of cases. The diagnostic significance of a fasting glucose concentration of greater than 7.0 mmol/L is of comparable diagnostic significance to a two hour post glucose load concentration of 11.1 mmol/L or more. Further evidence to support a lowering of the fasting glucose concentration for diagnosis came from studies that showed an increased risk of both microvascular and macrovascular disease in individuals with fasting values of 7.0 mmol/L or more, even if they had a normal two hour glucose concentration following a glucose load.

The ADA published its most recent recommendations for the diagnosis of DM in 1997, and much of the content of their report was accepted and incorporated into the WHO guidance. However, the US recommendations advocate the use of fasting glucose concentrations *alone* for diagnosis, without the need for performance of the OGTT for clinical purposes. The WHO recommendations favour the two hour post glucose load value as the more discriminatory, although accepting that for epidemiological studies, it may be more practical to use fasting values. The fundamental problem in the use of fasting glucose concentrations alone for diagnosis, is that, by definition, impaired glucose tolerance (IGT) cannot be diagnosed. A more practical problem is that it is frequently difficult to ascertain whether an individual is truly fasting.

The ADA and WHO criteria also differ in the use of the OGTT for the diagnosis of gestational DM. The WHO recommends that the procedure described above be followed for all individuals, including those who are pregnant. The ADA recommendations, whilst accepting that the OGTT performed with a 75 g glucose load identifies more pregnancies with maternal or perinatal complications associated with high plasma glucose concentrations, retain the 50 g glucose load OGTT, which was for many years to screen all pregnant women for gestational DM in the USA.

## THE STATES OF IMPAIRED GLUCOSE REGULATION: IMPAIRED FASTING GLYCAEMIA AND IMPAIRED GLUCOSE TOLERANCE

Impaired glucose tolerance (IGT) was first introduced as a category of glucose intolerance in the 1985 WHO guidelines; there is now considerable evidence that individuals so diagnosed are at increased risk of developing both DM and cardiovascular disease. The current WHO criteria recognise a further category of impaired glucose handling, namely impaired fasting glycaemia (IFG), which is also associated with an increased risk of DM and macrovascular disease.

Both IFG and IGT are now considered to be stages in the development of disordered carbohydrate metabolism and intermediate states between normal glucose homeostasis and DM. They should be viewed as at-risk categories for the development of DM and cardiovascular disease, rather than distinct clinical entities.

## AETIOLOGY OF IFG AND IGT

The factors that determine blood glucose concentration in the fasted state and two hours after a standard glucose load are different. Fasting blood glucose concentration is controlled by basal insulin secretion and hepatic glucose release, so abnormalities in either of these processes will lead to increased concentrations. In IFG, there are abnormalities of early insulin secretion and raised hepatic glucose output, the latter probably being related to altered hepatic sensitivity to insulin.

Following ingestion of a glucose load, the normal metabolic response is for glucose release from the liver to be suppressed and for increased insulin secretion to stimulate insulin-mediated glucose uptake by muscle and liver. In IGT, the major metabolic defect is peripheral resistance to insulin. This results in less efficient handling of a glucose load.

These two categories of impaired glucose handling will therefore identify different populations, both of which are 'at-risk' for development of DM. Individuals can have IFG, IGT or both, and those demonstrating combined IGT and IFG are at the greatest risk. IGT is more prevalent than IFG in most populations studied so far and is more strongly associated with cardiovascular risk.

## FUTURE DEVELOPMENTS
The report of a Consensus Workshop in 2002, convened by the International Diabetes Federation to review information relating to IFG and IGT, made several recommendations, which are likely to lead to further modifications to the way individuals with IFG and/or IGT, are identified, advised and, possibly, treated. Included in the recommendations are:

- a review of the diagnostic thresholds for all categories of glucose intolerance

- regular review of subjects with IFG and IGT, with reinforcement of lifestyle advice

- therapy with hypoglycaemic agents should be considered if lifestyle advice fails

- assessment of the value of plasma glucose measurements as part of cardiovascular risk assessment

- current and future intervention trials in IFG and IGT should focus on cardiovascular disease outcomes as well as progression to diabetes.

There is no doubt that the diagnostic criteria for DM and the states of impaired glucose regulation will continue to be modified, as knowledge and evidence of the association between precise concentrations of biochemical markers and the likelihood of development of the long-term complications grows.

# FURTHER READING

American Diabetes Association. Report of the expert committee on the diagnosis and classification of diabetes mellitus. Diabetes Care 1997; **20:** 1183-97.

American Diabetes Association. Diagnosis and classification of diabetes mellitus. Diabetes Care 2004; **27:** S5-S10.

Alberti KGMM, Zimmet PZ. Definition, diagnosis and classification of diabetes mellitus and its complications. Part 1: Diagnosis and classification of diabetes mellitus. Provisional report of a WHO consultation. Diabetic Med 1998; **15:** 539-53.

International Diabetes Federation IGT/IFG Consensus Statement. Impaired glucose tolerance and impaired fasting glycaemia: the current status on definition and intervention. Diabetic Med 2002; **19:** 708-23.

Lamb EJ, Day AP. New diagnostic criteria for diabetes mellitus: are we any further forward? Ann Clin Biochem 2000; **37:** 588-92.

World Health Organisation. Diabetes Mellitus: Report of a WHO Study Group. Geneva: World Health Organisation, 1985 (Technical Report Series 727).

## CLINICAL CASES

### GLYCOSURIA

A 30 year old man complained to his family doctor of a 3-4 month history of lethargy and generalised aching. His only medication was sodium valproate for epilepsy, although he had not had a fit for over five years. Examination of a random urine sample using a strip test in surgery revealed:

    glucose  +
    protein  0
    ketones  +

A venous sample, taken at the same time and analysed at the local hospital laboratory, had a plasma glucose concentration of 8.3 mmol/L. An OGTT was arranged:

| Time (min) | Plasma glucose (mmol/L) | Glycosuria |
|---|---|---|
| 0 | 5.2 | 0 |
| 60 | 14.3 | ++ |
| 120 | 7.0 | 0 |

Despite the patient's having glycosuria the OGTT was normal, excluding diabetes.

*POINTS:*

1. Urinary glucose values cannot be used for the diagnosis of DM according to the WHO or NDDG criteria.

2. The renal threshold for glucose displays wide inter-individual variation.

3. Certain drugs, e.g. sodium valproate, can give a false positive result on urine Ketostix® analysis for ketones.

### IMPAIRED GLUCOSE TOLERANCE

A 55 year old man was referred to the diabetes clinic following a well-patient clinic review by his family doctor at which he was noted to have + glycosuria on urinalysis (by enzyme reagent strip). He did not complain of any osmotic symptoms. He weighed 90 kg, with a body mass index (BMI) of 31 kg/m². He was an ex-smoker, having given up cigarettes two years previously. His hypertension was being treated with a β-blocker (atenolol 100 mg/day).

Blood tests taken by the family doctor showed a random glucose concentration of 9.0 mmol/L and cholesterol 7.8 mmol/L.

Results of a glucose tolerance test:

| Time (min) | Plasma glucose (mmol/L) | Glycosuria |
|---|---|---|
| 0 | 5.8 | 0 |
| 60 | 13.1 | ++ |
| 120 | 9.3 | 0 |

Other investigations included:

| Analyte | Result |
|---|---|
| Serum total cholesterol (mmol/L) | 8.8 |
| triglyceride (fasting) (mmol/L) | 3.7 |
| HDL cholesterol (mmol/L) | 1.01 |

The result of his OGTT shows that this patient has impaired glucose tolerance (WHO criteria). He was given dietary advice regarding a low fat, low refined sugar, weight reducing diet.

A follow up fasting blood sample was obtained three months later:

| Analyte | Result |
|---|---|
| Plasma glucose (mmol/L) | 5.9 |
| Serum fructosamine (μmol/L) | 250 |
| total cholesterol (mmol/L) | 8.0 |
| triglyceride (fasting) (mmol/L) | 3.6 |
| HDL cholesterol (mmol/L) | 1.05 |

He was commenced on lipid lowering medication (a fibrate).

*POINTS:*

1. Impaired glucose tolerance (IGT) carries a 2% per annum risk of progression to diabetes mellitus.

2. Unlike diabetes, IGT is not associated with microvascular (e.g. retinopathy, nephropathy) or neurological complications.

3. IGT is associated with an increased risk of macrovascular disease (and hence premature atherosclerotic cardiac disease). It is important to carry out a full cardio-vascular risk profile assessment on all patients with IGT.

4. Reaven's syndrome (or the metabolic syndrome) is an aggregation of several abnormalities that are associated with premature vascular disease. The features are: impaired glucose tolerance (including diabetes), hypertension, raised triglyceride and low HDL concentrations. At the heart of the syndrome is hyperinsulinism or, more strictly, insulin resistance. The syndrome is associated clinically with a high waist/hip ratio. It is unclear whether attempts to broaden the syndrome to include other abnormalities, e.g. raised urate, are justified.

# Chapter 4

# Management of diabetes

## DIET

The effect of diet in controlling the symptoms of diabetes is well documented throughout history. Early diets consisted mainly of carbohydrate and energy restriction and such diets were used in the treatment of type 1 diabetes before the discovery of insulin. Carbohydrate restriction was sometimes extreme (5-30 g/day) but while this did have some effect on the life expectancy of children with diabetes, it often resulted in their becoming extremely weak.

Following the introduction of insulin, restriction of food intake and particularly restriction of the carbohydrate content of the diet was the accepted practice for many years, and only recently has this view been relaxed. The concept of carbohydrate restriction was re-examined when it became obvious that cardiovascular disease (particularly coronary heart disease) was the major cause of mortality in the diabetic population. In any diet, the proportion of energy derived from protein tends to be fixed for financial reasons (protein is the most expensive part of a normal diet) and hence restricting carbohydrate inevitably leads to an increase in the amount derived from fat. It was clearly illogical to encourage a diet high in fat in patients with diabetes, who have a high cardiovascular morbidity and mortality.

## ENERGY INTAKE

The first step in determining the dietary requirements of a patient should be calculation of their energy needs. However, this is difficult because of the wide variation. In addition, the poorly controlled diabetic patient loses a variable amount of energy in the form of glucose in the urine. Historically, restriction of energy intake combined with losses in the urine led to undernutrition in children with type 1 diabetes, the so-called diabetic dwarf, and it is clear that children must be allowed a sufficient energy intake to grow normally, taking into account any lost in the urine. In contrast, many, if not the majority, of middle-aged and elderly patients with type 2 diabetes require less energy than their habitual intake. This is especially so when control is improved, urinary loss of glucose reduced, and hence more energy becomes available for storage.

Energy expenditure calculations, taking into account age, sex, and a broad category of physical activity (e.g. light or heavy) are available in the form of nomograms but are used less frequently than the more traditional (though less reliable) approaches, which include taking a dietary history and then calculating energy requirements.

*RESTRICTION OF ENERGY INTAKE*

This is important for many patients with diabetes, particularly type 2, who, if over-weight or obese, may require little else in the way of treatment. It also has a role to play in preventing excessive weight gain in patients treated with insulin.

The second step in devising a suitable diet is to determine the relative contributions of carbohydrate, protein and fat to the daily energy intake. Since protein intake varies little as a proportion of energy intake, the major decision centres on the relative proportions of fat and carbohydrate.

*RESTRICTION OF CARBOHYDRATE*

Carbohydrate is essential as an energy source. Diets containing 100 g of carbohydrate or more are required to prevent protein loss and the excessive metabolism of fat that occurs to provide energy in carbohydrate starvation.

Restriction of the total amount of carbohydrate in the diabetic diet is now of historical interest only but for two exceptions. First, some consistency in both the overall amount consumed during the day, and at particular times during the day, continues to be advised; this is less important with flexible insulin regimens, in which patients monitor their own blood glucose concentrations and can adjust their dose of insulin before a meal. Second, restriction of refined carbohydrate is advised to avoid the exaggerated swings in blood glucose concentration that can occur after consumption of mono- and disaccharides.

*THE HIGH CARBOHYDRATE DIET*

Several studies have shown no change in glycaemic control in comparisons of low and high carbohydrate diets, although an approximately equal number have shown some deterioration in control with high carbohydrate feeding. It is likely that the method of presentation of the carbohydrate is of importance *viz.* starch *versus* mono-saccharides. Generally, starch is present in fibre-containing food, which may slow the digestion and absorption of carbohydrate. Other forms of fibre, such as the gelatinous fibres, guar and pectin, clearly reduce postprandial glucose excursions but with the exception of pectin in marmalades, they exist solely as a dietary supplement.

*FAT*

Fat is essential in the diet only as a source of fat-soluble vitamins, most of which can be obtained from other sources, and to supply essential fatty acids. Fat provides 9 kcal/g as opposed to the 4 kcal/g provided by carbohydrate and protein, and thus supplies energy in a lesser bulk. This may once have been advantageous, though whether it remains so in the present day is debatable. Thus, it is relatively easy to consume 50% of the daily energy requirement as fat but rather more difficult to eat the volume of carbohydrate that will give 50% of energy needs, especially if this is to be taken from high fibre sources rather than the refined carbohydrates. Even with the recommendation of a high carbohydrate intake, however, it is difficult to get fat intake below 35-40% of daily energy intake.

*PROTEIN*
The diabetic diet should contain the normal recommended daily intake of protein, that is, 50-60 g/day for adult males and 40-50 g/day for females, which approximates to 10-15 % of the daily intake of energy.

## CURRENT RECOMMENDATIONS ON DIET FOR PATIENTS WITH DIABETES
In summary, the first step in the dietary management of diabetic patients is to estimate the amount of energy needed to help the patient towards their ideal body weight. There is no need for restriction of carbohydrate, as long as it is taken as complex carbohydrate. Indeed, an increase to 50% of total energy intake may have a beneficial effect upon control. Some restriction of mono- or disaccharides should persist wherever possible, except as treatment for hypoglycaemia or when illness necessitates this type of intake.

In the hope of reducing arterial disease, it is recommended that no more than 35% of total energy be derived from fat. This should be achieved primarily by reducing cooking and spreading fats, dairy products and meat and meat products. For palatability, about 50% of the remaining fat should be in the unsaturated form.

## ORAL AGENTS
Tablets for the treatment of diabetes have been available since the middle of the last century and have undoubtedly allowed some patients with type 2 diabetes to avoid treatment with insulin. However, long-term studies such as the United Kingdom Prospective Diabetes Study (UKPDS) have shown that type 2 diabetes is a progressive disorder in which the continuing decline in β cell function leads to a deterioration of glycaemic control with time. This is often seen clinically when patients progress from diet to tablets, and through combinations of tablets to insulin, as the years go by.

## SULPHONYLUREAS
Sulphonylureas are the most widely used oral agents for the treatment of type 2 diabetes. They have been used in clinical practice for more than 40 years and are of proven efficacy and safety, although many aspects of their mechanism of action remain incompletely understood.

*PHARMACOLOGY*

The active part of the drug molecule is a sulphonyl group linked to a ureide. The chemical groups that surround this essential core determine the properties of the various compounds, including their pathways of metabolism. It is important to appreciate the difference between the pharmacokinetic and pharmacodynamic profiles of the various sulphonylureas. Some, e.g. glibenclamide, have a short half-life in the circulation yet produce severely prolonged episodes of hypoglycaemia under certain conditions. There are many sulphonylureas on the market, and new ones continue to be developed with the aim of improving safety and reducing side-effects.

*MODE OF ACTION*

The mechanism by which sulphonylureas lower blood glucose has gradually emerged as our understanding of the pathogenesis of type 2 diabetes has become clearer. Both insulin resistance and diminished insulin secretion contribute to the pathogenesis and sulphonylureas may influence both of these processes.

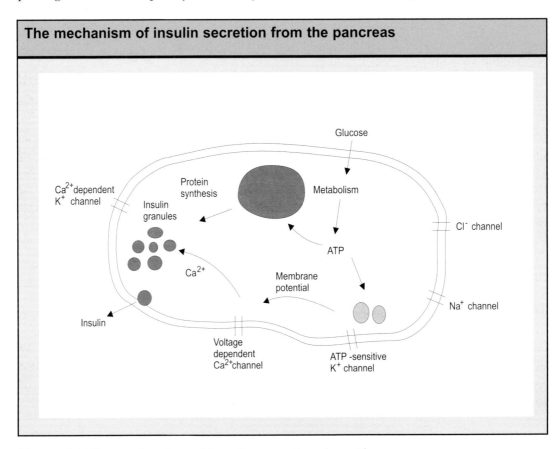

**The mechanism of insulin secretion from the pancreas**

Figure 4.1 The mechanism of insulin secretion from the pancreas

In early animal studies, a substantial body of evidence accumulated that the sulphonylureas act directly on the pancreas. It was clearly demonstrated that they cause a decrease in islet β cell granulation and in the insulin content of the pancreas. Similarly, in human studies, it was demonstrated with all the potent sulphonylureas that, following administration of the drug, blood glucose concentration is lowered through an increase in circulating insulin concentration. In these clinical studies, however, it was also apparent that although initially the lowering of blood glucose is accompanied by an enhanced insulin response, with prolonged treatment the improvement in blood glucose is maintained but insulin concentrations return to pre-treatment concentrations. This long-term effect was initially called the extra-pancreatic mechanism of action. More recently, appreciation of the concept of insulin resistance has lead to the conclusion that part of the mechanism of action of sulphonylureas is through an enhancement of sensitivity to insulin.

*CLINICAL USAGE*

The major use of sulphonylureas is in type 2 patients who are not grossly overweight but in whom dietary therapy alone does not produce near-normal glycaemia. In this situation, they are often used as monotherapy. Additionally, sulphonylureas may be used in combination with metformin in more obese patients who are not adequately controlled on metformin alone.

Sulphonylureas are not used in type 1 diabetes and hence are rarely used in children or adolescents, except when it is unclear which type of diabetes the patient has. In recent years, it has become more common to see type 2 diabetes in children and it is quite common to encounter clinical situations where the type of diabetes is unclear. For example, in a young teenager who is found to have a blood glucose concentration that is mildly raised but sufficiently to diagnose diabetes, it is often not clear whether they have type 2 diabetes or type 1 diabetes detected at a very early stage of the disease.

Sulphonylureas are not used in pregnancy since the drug crosses the placenta and causes fetal hyperinsulinism.

The use of sulphonylurea drugs in patients treated with insulin has been claimed to improve control and well-being. Any beneficial effect of a sulphonylurea in type 1 patients would depend upon a significant insulin sensitising effect of the drug. At best, this might be expected to reduce insulin requirements somewhat. However, the total daily dose of insulin varies so widely from patient to patient that it is difficult to prove this. There is probably no role for sulphonylureas in this situation.

The accumulated clinical experience of using sulphonylureas has confirmed that significant side-effects are encountered only rarely. Although many side-effects have been described, most are exceedingly rare and date from the early days of treatment, when dosage was often inappropriately high. Hypoglycaemia and weight gain are the major side effects of clinical relevance (*see Figure 4.2*).

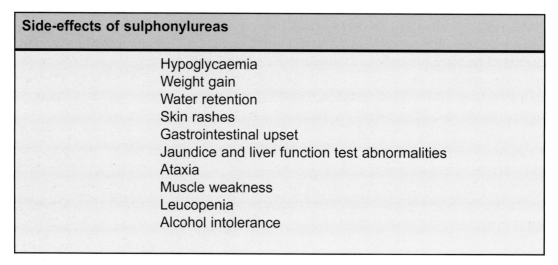

**Side-effects of sulphonylureas**

Hypoglycaemia
Weight gain
Water retention
Skin rashes
Gastrointestinal upset
Jaundice and liver function test abnormalities
Ataxia
Muscle weakness
Leucopenia
Alcohol intolerance

**Figure 4.2 Side-effects of sulphonylureas**

Hypoglycaemia, although relatively uncommon, is still a significant complication of the use of sulphonylureas. It often occurs when treatment is started and becomes less frequent with continuing use. Mild attacks are probably more frequent than is appreciated by medical staff. They tend to occur before the midday or evening meals, and are most likely to occur with the more potent or longer acting sulphonylureas such as chlorpropamide and glibenclamide.

Severe hypoglycaemic attacks with coma are seen in elderly patients who may be in a poor state of nutrition or prone to self-neglect. Declining renal function often plays a part in reducing excretion of the drug or an active metabolite. In addition, those who take alcohol in place of a normal meal are particularly susceptible to hypoglycaemia. Severe attacks may be prolonged and refractory to treatment and fatalities have been reported. Very high plasma concentrations of sulphonylurea have been found in such cases and a failure of metabolism or excretion could well be an important factor.

A severe hypoglycaemic attack due to sulphonylureas is a medical emergency. It is still not always appreciated that treatment of sulphonylurea-induced hypoglycaemic coma should take place in hospital. Even when the patient gets to hospital, casualty officers are so used to the quick response to intravenous glucose in patients with hypoglycaemic coma from insulin that they may fail to distinguish sulphonylurea-induced from insulin-induced hypoglycaemia.

High circulating concentrations of both sulphonylureas and insulin can be measured. A patient with hypoglycaemia on sulphonylurea therapy is hypoglycaemic from *endogenous* insulin. Furthermore, the high concentrations of insulin will persist as long as the sulphonylurea is present. The problem is compounded in that the only means of treating hypoglycaemia and raising blood glucose concentration is by the use of an insulin secretagogue, either glucose or glucagon, and these must be used in a situation where the β cells are sensitised to secretory effects by the sulphonylurea. The continued stimulus to insulin production, and insulin-sensitising effects of the circulating sulphonylurea will persist until the latter is metabolised or excreted. Relapse into hypoglycaemia following initial treatment and possibly some physical recovery is common and predictable, and almost inevitable if glucagon or only a bolus of glucose is given. The correct treatment of severe sulphonylurea-induced hypoglycaemia is a glucose infusion that must be maintained until the sulphonylurea is cleared.

Sulphonylurea-induced hypoglycaemia may present as a stroke that is completely reversible with appropriate treatment of the hypoglycaemia. Hypoglycaemia in the elderly presenting as a hemiparesis is sufficiently common to warrant blood glucose measurement in any diabetic patient arriving in an Accident and Emergency Department with an apparent stroke.

Weight gain is, in practice, the most frequent side-effect of treatment with sulphonylureas. The precise mechanism remains unclear. All patients whose glycaemic control improves without dietary modification would be expected to gain weight. In the uncontrolled state, energy is lost as glucose in the urine that then becomes available for storage as control improves. This is not the complete explanation, however, as weight gain often exceeds that which might be expected from this mechanism. An additional factor may be that patients have a more relaxed approach to diet when they perceive that tablets are the main agent of treatment.

It is well recognised that chlorpropamide potentiates the effect of antidiuretic hormone on renal tubules. Indeed, this effect has been used as the basis for treating some patients with diabetes insipidus with this drug. In patients with diabetes mellitus, it may be difficult to detect this unwanted side-effect, which can lead to hyponatraemia and cause major problems such as seizure or coma. These seem to be more likely to occur in patients simultaneously taking a thiazide diuretic.

Chlorpropamide is now little used in type 2 diabetes, mainly because of the risk of hypoglycaemia, but also because it can cause water retention: both side-effects tend to be difficult to treat because the drug has a long half-life (approximately 36 h).

*DRUG INTERACTIONS (Figure 4.3)*
Sulphonylureas are transported in the plasma bound to albumin, and any drug that shares this transport mechanism may potentiate the effects of a sulphonylurea by displacing it from the protein. Aspirin, sulphonamides and trimethoprim have all been implicated in severe sulphonylurea-induced hypoglycaemia. In a similar manner, the introduction of sulphonylurea therapy may have implications for patients on other drugs that can bind to albumin, for example, warfarin.

| Drug interactions with sulphonylureas |
| --- |
| Class interactions |
|     Coumarins |
|     Monoamine oxidase inhibitors |
|     Sulphonamides |
|     Tetracyclines |
|   |
| Specific drug interactions |
|     Alcohol |
|     Azapropazone |
|     Chloramphenicol |
|     Cimetidine |
|     Co-trimoxazole |
|     Cyclophosphamide |
|     Miconazole |
|     Rifampicin |
|     Salicylate |
|     Sulphinpyrazone |
|     Trimethoprim |

**Figure 4.3 Drug interactions with sulphonylureas**

BIGUANIDES
Metformin (dimethylbiguanide) is the only biguanide in common use. The earlier biguanides, phenformin and buformin, have largely been withdrawn from clinical use because of the risk of lactic acidosis. The precise mode of action of biguanides has proved difficult to elicit and it seems likely that at least three processes are affected.

First, there is considerable evidence from studies in animals that biguanides inhibit hepatic gluconeogenesis. Such evidence is difficult to obtain in man, although in normal man, decreased lactate uptake and glucose output by the liver has been reported, and during euglycaemic clamping, metformin enhances the inhibition of hepatic glucose output by insulin. Second, measurement of arterio-venous differences across the human forearm has shown increased peripheral uptake of glucose with biguanides. Third, decreased glucose absorption from the gut has been observed in animals and man following biguanide administration.

More recent studies have shown an effect of metformin on insulin receptors and enhancement of post-receptor metabolism of glucose, and this latter finding, in conjunction with the observation that metformin lowers blood glucose concentrations without increasing insulin concentrations, has led to the conclusion that metformin acts primarily by increasing the sensitivity of liver and muscle to insulin.

*THERAPEUTIC USE*

Metformin is used in the treatment of type 2 diabetes in three distinct situations. It acts directly upon metabolism to improve blood glucose concentrations, and does not stimulate insulin secretion: indeed, lower insulin concentrations result from reductions in plasma glucose concentrations. Hence, patients are less likely to gain weight with metformin treatment and for this reason it is often used as a monotherapy in obese patients with type 2 diabetes. An additional benefit is that metformin has an anorectic effect, which also makes weight loss rather than weight gain more likely with its use.

When secondary resistance to a sulphonylurea develops, it is sometimes possible to re-establish control by the use of metformin in combination with the sulphonylurea.

The use of biguanides in combination with insulin is more controversial. In type 2 diabetic patients who require insulin, giving metformin may allow control of blood glucose with a lower dosage of insulin, owing to the insulin sensitising effect of metformin, although whether this is a goal worth attaining is debatable. In practice, there is rather better evidence for the use of metformin to restrict weight gain in obese patients requiring insulin.

*SIDE-EFFECTS*

Side-effects of metformin are common: diarrhoea is the most troublesome. In general, this is an under-recognised side-effect of the drug, and a number of patients needlessly undergo investigation of the large bowel because of it. Other side-effects include anorexia, nausea and vomiting, weakness, vague malaise and a metallic taste in the mouth.

Serious toxic effects are rare with conservative dosage. Ketonuria is usually attributable to starvation ketosis as a result of anorexia and a low carbohydrate intake. An increased carbohydrate intake is said to reverse it.

One toxic effect is of major importance: soon after the introduction of the first biguanide, phenformin, the occurrence of a severe non-ketotic metabolic acidosis in diabetic patients was reported. The risk is, however, lower with metformin, and of the few cases of lactic acidosis during metformin therapy that have been reported, nearly all reflect inappropriate prescribing. However, some cases of metformin-induced lactic acidosis may be being overlooked, particularly in the situation where a diabetic patient on metformin has a myocardial infarction or severe infection.

### CONTRAINDICATIONS

It is sensible to avoid prescribing metformin when patients have an associated illness that affects either peripheral lactate production or hepatic lactate clearance. These disorders include ischaemic heart disease and chronic pulmonary disease.

Metformin undergoes renal clearance and accumulation of the drug occurs if renal function is impaired. For this reason, metformin is contraindicated in patients with declining renal function. Most reports of metformin-induced lactic acidosis have been in patients with renal failure who were maintained on metformin.

Although contraindications should be sought before starting treatment, they may develop during treatment. Some will be readily apparent and necessitate changing therapy. Others, such as declining renal function, particularly with age, can be more insidious and some form of monitoring is necessary. Measurement of creatinine clearance annually is impractical but an elevated plasma creatinine concentration, which usually reflects a considerable reduction in renal function, should be a clear indication for withdrawing metformin. However, there is no consensus on the concentration of creatinine that should lead to the withdrawal of metformin or is a contraindication to its use. Some diabetologists allow plasma creatinine concentration to rise to 200 μmol/L before withdrawing the drug, although this seems to be unnecessarily courting disaster; many practitioners do not prescribe metformin if a patient's plasma creatinine concentration is elevated to any extent.

Recently, there has been interest in using metformin in some forms of liver disease, particularly associated with fatty liver and insulin resistance. Since metformin has profound effects upon metabolism in the liver this should be done with extreme caution.

## ALPHA-GLUCOSIDASE INHIBITORS

There are a number of alpha-glucosidase inhibitors on the market, of which the best known in Europe is acarbose.

Alpha-glucosidase inhibitors inhibit digestion of complex carbohydrates through enzyme inhibition, leading to delayed absorption of the monosaccharide. In normal people, addition of acarbose to a sucrose load decreases the absorption of its mono-saccharides by up to 40%. In patients with type 2 diabetes, glucose tolerance is improved, while in patients with type 1 diabetes, post-prandial rises in blood glucose are reduced and insulin requirements are decreased by about one-third. It is important to appreciate that hypoglycaemia in patients treated with acarbose, which occurs only in combination with oral agents or insulin, will not respond to oral mono- or disaccharides.

In clinical practice, results rarely seem as good as those obtained under the more rigid conditions of clinical trials. At best, acarbose reduces $HbA_{1c}$ by less than 1% and its use tends to be limited by side-effects. The major, and most frequent, side-effect is flatulence, which results from fermentation of unabsorbed carbohydrate by colonic bacteria.

## POSTPRANDIAL GLUCOSE REGULATORS

Repaglinide was the first in a new class of oral hypoglycaemic agents described as post-prandial glucose regulators. It is a carbamoylmethyl benzoic acid derivative, with structural similarities to the non-sulphonylurea side-chain of the sulphonylurea glibenclamide. A second drug in this class, nateglinide, is a phenylalanine derivative.

Both repaglinide and nateglinide are insulin secretagogues, acting by inhibition of the ATP-dependent potassium ion channel on pancreatic β cells. This results in depolarisation of the membrane, influx of calcium, and stimulation of insulin secretion. Repaglinide binds to the sulphonylurea receptor and to a specific site on the β cell membrane.

Both drugs are short acting insulin secretagogues. Repaglinide is absorbed rapidly and eliminated rapidly, with both the $T_{(max)}$ and the $T_{½}$ being approximately 40-60 min. Consequently, there is a short insulinotrophic action, resulting in a reduction in post-prandial glucose excursions.

Post-prandial glucose regulators are effective in lowering fasting blood glucose concentrations and glycated haemoglobin, either when used alone or in combination with other oral hypoglycaemic agents. Studies have been performed in combination with metformin, thiazolidinediones and insulin with promising results. Clearly, since they are insulin secretagogues, there is no logical case to be made for using them in combination with sulphonylureas.

Metabolism of repaglinide is by the hepatic cytochrome P450 enzymes. Other drugs that have effects upon the cytochrome P450 system interact with repaglinide. The anti-fungal agent ketoconazole inhibits this system, while rifampicin, barbiturates, and carbamazepine induce the P450 3A4 isoenzyme, thus enhancing the metabolism of repaglinide. Corticosteroids and cyclosporin are also reported to inhibit its metabolism.

THIAZOLIDINEDIONES

These drugs are insulin sensitizers, that is, they reduce insulin resistance without having a direct effect upon insulin secretion. As such, the launch of the first in the class, troglitazone was greeted with great acclaim, since it represented an entirely new class of drug aimed at one of the major aspects of the pathogenesis of diabetes, particularly in the overweight and obese. Although introduced in several countries, it was very soon withdrawn in the UK, and subsequently in the USA, because of fears over hepatotoxicity. More recently, successors to troglitazone have been introduced, namely rosiglitazone and pioglitazone.

Thiazolidinediones lower blood glucose and insulin concentrations in a variety of animal models of diabetes and in patients with type 2 diabetes. They potentiate insulin-induced glucose uptake into peripheral tissues and lower hepatic glucose output. At the molecular level, these drugs appear to work directly or indirectly on specific receptors in the cell nucleus, the peroxisome proliferator-activated receptors gamma 1 & 2 (PPARs).

Because they are insulin sensitizers, both rosiglitazone and pioglitazone are of value in the treatment of obese patients with type 2 diabetes. It follows from their mode of action that their greatest use might be in the early stages of type 2 diabetes, when insulin secretory reserve is being compromised by increased demand because of insulin resistance. They might also be indicated to reduce insulin requirements in obese patients treated with insulin. Somewhat illogically, however, the licence for these drugs in the UK was initially only for combination therapy with either a sulphonylurea or metformin. This can result in patients poorly controlled on sulphonylurea or metformin having one of these drugs withdrawn and a thiazolidinedione substituted. Often in this situation, the more appropriate change would be to introduce insulin. It is likely that the licence will be modified to extend the indications, particularly as monotherapy and, perhaps, for impaired glucose tolerance. However, their use in combination with insulin is specifically contraindicated.

All drugs of this class require 3-6 months before their full impact upon blood glucose concentration and $HbA_{1c}$ is apparent. Preliminary studies with both rosiglitazone and pioglitazone suggest that the hepatotoxicity reported with troglitazone is not a class effect but is probably related to the side-chain substitution. However, there is a requirement for monitoring liver function and discontinuation of therapy if plasma aminotransferase activities exceed three times the upper limits of their reference ranges.

Side-effects are a significant problem. They occur in 2-5% of patients and include anaemia and peripheral oedema. Weight gain is a consequence of the mode of action: increased sensitivity of adipocytes to insulin inevitably leads to greater fat deposition and decreased lipolysis.

## INSULIN

Insulin is used in the treatment of type 1 diabetes from diagnosis and in type 2 diabetes when oral therapy fails. A large number of insulin preparations exist, which can be broadly categorised into short acting, long acting, and pre-mixed insulins. Making a distinction between intermediate acting and long acting insulins is outdated. Although for many years, insulin was derived from animals (cattle and pigs), recombinant DNA technology has made 'human' insulin widely available and this is now almost exclusively used.

The aims of treatment with insulin are no different from the goals of dietary modification or treatment with oral agents, that is, to achieve and maintain blood glucose concentrations as near to normal as possible without inducing the disabling side-effect of hypoglycaemia. This first objective is more pressing in young patients with type 1 diabetes, who are faced with upwards of 30 years with diabetes during which there is a high risk of developing complications. The second may be more of a concern in elderly patients without diabetic complications who live alone.

The general principle of insulin treatment is to give sufficient, at appropriate times, to control blood glucose concentration. However, there is no fixed replacement dose of insulin as there is, for example, of thyroxine in hypothyroidism. In other words, both the total daily dose of insulin and the distribution of this between injections has to be tailored to meet the individual patient's requirements.

There are two main regimens for insulin delivery: these are twice daily combinations of short and long acting insulins, and the basal-bolus regimen. The former is used extensively in type 2 diabetes; the latter is used principally in type 1 diabetes, particularly from adolescence onward, although there is considerable overlap in their usage.

A regimen of twice daily mixtures of short and long acting insulins, for example Actrapid® or Humulin S® with the isophane insulins Insulatard® or Humulin I®, taken before breakfast and the evening meal, is designed such that the short acting insulin covers breakfast and evening meal and the longer acting insulin covers the glucose provided by the midday meal and provides an overnight supply of insulin. Mixtures of short and long acting insulin can be of any relative proportions: pre-mixed preparations are available, of which the most widely used are a 50/50 mixture and one with 30% short acting and 70% long acting.

The basal-bolus regimen was devised in the hope of achieving better glycaemic control throughout the day and night by attempting to mimic 'normal' physiology. People who do not have diabetes secrete insulin in response to meals and snacks. In the basal-bolus regimen, an attempt is made to imitate this by injecting quick acting insulin three times daily before meals and a long acting insulin before going to bed to provide insulin during sleep and on waking. The advent of pen injection devices had made such regimens more acceptable to patients. It is debatable whether they produce better control of blood glucose than conventional regimens but they do give greater freedom of lifestyle, particularly with regard to the timing of meals, which is enjoyed by patients. Other regimens include continuous sub-cutaneous insulin infusion and the DAFNE regimen (Dose Adjustment for Normal Eating) but at present, these are appropriate for only small numbers of patients.

INSULIN ANALOGUES

Knowledge of the genetic code for human insulin has allowed the production of a series of insulin analogues. An obstacle to compliance and control with human insulin is the necessity for insulin to be injected 20-40 minutes before eating. This is due to insulin molecules forming dimers and hexamers at the site of injection. Time and dilution at the injection site is required before insulin disassociates into monomers and can be absorbed across capillary walls. This slows absorption and prolongs the action of insulin. Two short acting insulin analogues have been produced and marketed that have specific advantages over standard human insulin. These have modifications to the chemical structure that alter the association and disassociation of the molecules into dimers and hexamers. Insulin lyspro (Humalog®) is an insulin in which the lysine-proline sequence at B28 and B29 is reversed; insulin aspart (NovoRapid®) is an analogue in which aspartate replaces proline at position B28 (*see Figure 4.4*). Both are rapidly absorbed from injection sites and can, therefore, be given at the start of a meal.

## Short acting insulin analogues

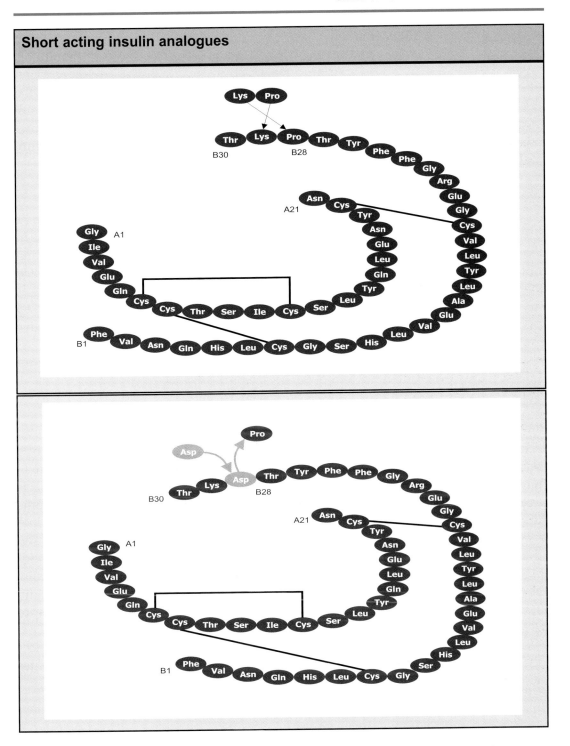

Figure 4.4 Short acting insulin analogues lyspro (top) and aspart (bottom)

To date, one long acting insulin analogue has been produced: insulin Glargine®. This produces a steady background release of insulin and relatively constant circulating concentrations of insulin, thus mimicking the normal physiological supply.

The aim of treatment is to minimise the risk of long-term diabetic complications through good control of blood glucose concentrations. The major obstacle to achieving this goal is hypoglycaemia. There is clear evidence that hypoglycaemia becomes more likely the lower the $HbA_{1c}$ concentration, and there is also evidence that tight control of blood glucose concentration leads to a loss of appreciation of impending hypoglycaemia.

## ASSESSMENT OF GLYCAEMIC CONTROL

Assessment of glycaemic control is important for two reasons. Glycaemic control indicates the level of risk for the development of complications to which the patient is exposed. It also indicates how regimens can be altered in order to improve control and hence reduce risk.

Overall blood glucose control is best assessed by measurement of a glycated protein (usually haemoglobin) although some indication may be obtained from patients' records of home blood glucose monitoring. Urine testing for glucose is of little value in the assessment of glycaemic control although it may, understandably, be preferred by patients.

When overall glucose control, as assessed by glycated protein measurement, is unsatisfactory, home blood glucose monitoring gives an indication of how treatment may be altered. This is most useful in patients treated with insulin, as these results should indicate which insulin injection should be altered in order to improve control.

In summary, assessment of glycaemic control is a two-step process: first, is overall control satisfactory (using a glycated protein measurement) and, if not, how can it be improved? Options for the latter include a change of regimen e.g. from diet to tablets or tablets to insulin in a patient with type 2 diabetes (usually based on measurement of $HbA_{1c}$) or adjustment of the insulin regimen (usually based on blood glucose monitoring).

What are the goals of treatment? Simply that blood glucose control, reflected in glycated protein measurement, should be as good as possible. The results of both the Diabetes Control and Complications Trial (DCCT) and the UKPDS suggested that the effect of control upon the risk of development of complications is a continuum and thus that progressive benefit should accrue with progressive reduction of a raised glycated protein concentration. Of course, in an ideal world, treatment would allow the attainment and maintenance of normoglycaemia at all times. In practice, this is rarely possible, particularly for patients with type 1 diabetes, in whom efforts to achieve excellent control inevitably increase the risk of hypoglycaemia. In patients with type 2 diabetes, the risk of hypoglycaemia is much less, although they may encounter problems with weight gain.

## OTHER BIOCHEMICAL ASPECTS OF CONTROL

In addition to blood glucose concentration, a number of other biochemical variables are important in the management of diabetes. The development of ketonuria is an important warning sign in diabetic patients at times of intercurrent illness. Meters are currently available that will measure plasma ketones, or more specifically 3-hydroxybutyrate, as well as glucose, but the majority of patients still use Ketostix® testing of urine.

In the clinic, the detection of microalbuminuria before the stage of Albustix® positive albuminuria is reached indicates early renal involvement and may prompt the introduction of specific therapies e.g. ACE inhibitors, which may slow the progression of disease. In established renal disease, measurement of serum creatinine concentration will be required.

Although glucose concentration is related to the development of microvascular complications, there is considerably less evidence that glucose plays a major part in the macrovascular complications that result in so much morbidity and mortality. Assessment of circulating lipids is therefore important, including measurement of total cholesterol, triglycerides, and HDL-cholesterol. Although it is fairly clear that lipid abnormalities do not alone explain the excess mortality from atheroma in the diabetic population, nevertheless all the evidence is that patients with diabetes gain at least as much benefit as the general population from cholesterol lowering. With regard to triglycerides, the situation is less clear. Hypertriglyceridaemia is a frequent feature of poor glycaemic control. Effective treatment of the diabetes reduces circulating triglyceride concentrations. In practice, however, one encounters many patients with raised serum triglycerides and sub-optimal control in whom there is little prospect of improving glycaemic control. However, it is clearly important to target patients with triglyceride concentrations that put them at risk of pancreatitis (> 10 mmol/L). There is also evidence of benefit from triglyceride lowering in those in whom a high triglyceride concentration is accompanied by a low HDL-cholesterol concentration (< 1.0 mmol/L).

# FURTHER READING

Asplund K, Wiholm BE, Lithner F. Glibenclamide-associated hypoglycaemia: A report of 57 cases. Diabetologia 1983; **24:** 412-7.

Banting FG, Best CH, Collip JB *et al.* Pancreatic extracts in the treatment of diabetes mellitus. Can Med Ass J 1922; **12:** 141-6.

Brange J, Ribel U, Hansen JE *et al.* Monomeric insulins obtained by protein engineering and their medical implications. Nature 1988; **333:** 679-82.

Diabetes Prevention Program Research Group. Reduction in the incidence of type 2 diabetes and lifestyle intervention or metformin. N Engl J Med 2002; **346:** 393-403.

Lean MEJ, James WPT. Prescription of diabetic diets in the 1980s. Lancet 1986; **I:** 723-5.

Owens DR, Zinman B, Bolli GB. Insulins today and beyond. Lancet 2001; **358:** 739-46.

Owens DR, Griffiths S. Insulin Glargine (Lantus). Int J Clin Pract 2002; **56:** 460-6.

Leatherdale BA, Panesar RK, Singh G *et al.* Improvement in glucose tolerance due to *Momordica charantia* (karela). Br Med J 1981; **282:** 1823-4.

UKPDS. UK Prospective Study of therapies of maturity-onset diabetes. 1. Effect of diet, sulphonylurea, insulin or biguanide therapy on fasting plasma glucose and body weight over 1 year. Diabetologia 1983; **24:** 404-11.

## CLINICAL CASES

### CHANGING INSULIN REGIMEN FROM TWICE DAILY TO FOUR TIMES DAILY INSULIN

A seventeen year-old Caucasian male was diagnosed as having type 1 diabetes, following a short history (two weeks) of excessive thirst, polyuria, nocturia and increasing tiredness. His random plasma glucose concentration on presentation was 17.4 mmol/L.

He was commenced on a twice daily regimen of pre-mixed insulin and became stabilised on a dose of 20 units mane, 14 units nocte. Twelve months after diagnosis control remained good as evidenced by home glucose monitoring and an $HbA_{1c}$ of 7.0%.

Over the following 12 months, however, his glycaemic control deteriorated. His home glucose monitoring revealed frequent values of 12-18 mmol/L, particularly in the afternoon and early evening. On review in the diabetic clinic, random capillary plasma glucose concentration was 12.1 mmol/L and $HbA_{1c}$ 9.8%. He also reported that he had begun experiencing neuroglycopaenic symptoms of hypoglycaemia, namely tremors, sweating and light-headedness. These occurred at a frequency of 1-2 such episodes per week, often being associated with exercise. The patient was an amateur athlete (an 800 m and 1500 m runner) and found control particularly difficult on race and training days, despite reducing his insulin dose at these times.

In order to allow him greater flexibility in altering his insulin dose in relation to anticipated activity, his regimen was altered to one of four insulin injections per day, namely a dose of short acting insulin before each meal (breakfast, lunch, and evening meal) plus a dose of long acting insulin at night, and he was asked to perform home glucose monitoring four times daily. The doses of short acting insulin were reduced by ~ 2 units on race and training days.

After six months on this regimen (typically, quick acting insulin 10U, 10U, 10U with 12U of long acting insulin at night, with the patient making adjustments based on his own home glucose monitoring and expected exercise), his home blood glucose measurements were mainly in the range 4-9 mmol/L, with no discernible pattern of high or low values; his $HbA_{1c}$ was 7.5%.

1. Four times per day insulin regimens are often favoured by highly motivated patients and those whose lifestyles feature significant regular exercise or physical activity.

2. Newly diagnosed patients with type 1 diabetes often experience a 'honeymoon period' in the initial stages of insulin treatment during which good diabetic control is established and maintained on modest doses of insulin. This phase commonly lasts for 1-2 years, following which control gradually deteriorates unless insulin dosage is increased.

3. The choice of a quick acting insulin now includes rapid acting insulin analogues such as insulin aspart (NovoRapid) and lyspro (Humalog). These insulins are more convenient for young people because they can be given immediately before a meal, and, because they are rapidly absorbed, they have a greater impact on post-prandial glucose excursions compared with human Actrapid or Humulin S insulin.

## CHANGING FROM TABLETS TO INSULIN

A 52-year-old-man attended the diabetes clinic for review. He had been diagnosed with diabetes eight years earlier and was a regular attender. At diagnosis, his weight was 85 kg and BMI 30 kg/m$^2$. Initial treatment had been with an energy-restricted diet, and six months after diagnosis, he had reduced his weight to 82.5 kg. A year after diagnosis, his weight had returned to 85 kg and metformin was added to his dietary treatment. Control was satisfactory on metformin for 18 months but then deteriorated. He was given a small dose of a sulphonylurea. Control improved initially but he subsequently required increasing doses of a sulphonylurea in an attempt to control his diabetes.

On this occasion control was once again unsatisfactory. The table summarises glycaemic control and treatment changes over the eight years following diagnosis.

| Time | Weight (kg) | Glucose (mmol/L) | HbA$_{1c}$ (%) | Treatment change |
|---|---|---|---|---|
| Diagnosis | 85.0 | 17.2 | 10.2 | Energy restriction |
| + 6 months | 82.5 | 9.8 | 6.7 | |
| + 12 months | 85.2 | 15.8 | 8.0 | Add metformin 500 mg t.d.s |
| + 2.5 years | 83.4 | 14.0 | 8.2 | Add gliclazide 40 mg daily |
| + 3 years | 86.0 | 10.9 | 7.2 | Increase to 80 mg daily |
| + 3.5 years | 86.5 | 7.2 | 6.5 | |
| + 4 years | 86.7 | 8.1 | 6.7 | |
| + 5 years | 84.3 | 14.2 | 7.4 | Increase to 80 mg twice daily |
| + 5.5 years | 85.0 | 12.1 | 7.8 | Increase to 160 mg a.m. 80 mg p.m. |
| + 6 years | 83.3 | 9.0 | 8.4 | Increase metformin to 850 mg t.d.s. |
| + 7 years | 82.0 | 9.2 | 8.9 | Increase gliclazide to 160 mg twice daily |
| + 8 years | 80.1 | 12.2 | 9.5 | ? |

*POINTS*

1. This man presumably has type 2 diabetes although there is not a great deal of evidence that he ever responded satisfactorily to standard treatment for type 2 diabetes. The results six months after diagnosis and at 3½ and 4 years suggest some response to diet and subsequently, the addition of a secretagogue.

2. When control is poor despite a small dose of sulphonylurea, it is debatable whether increasing the dose of the sulphonylurea is worthwhile. There is little evidence for a dose response relationship in this situation.

3. It is often salutary to review results over preceding attendances. It is clear that glycaemic control in this man has been poor for some time.

4. Type 2 diabetes tends to worsen with time and in this man, who was only 52 years old at diagnosis, it is very unlikely that he will get through the rest of his life without needing insulin. Thus the decision here is not whether he needs insulin but when, and the inescapable conclusion from his accumulated results is that he should probably have been started on insulin some time ago.

# Chapter 5

# Hyperglycaemic comas

## INTRODUCTION

Diabetic ketoacidosis (DKA) and hyperosmolar non-ketotic coma (HONK) remain significant causes of mortality in type 1 and type 2 diabetes. While the pathogenesis of DKA is relatively well understood, that of HONK is less so. Clinically, hyperglycaemia, and the symptoms and signs which result from the raised glucose concentration, is the factor common in their presentation and, while the presence of significant ketosis and acidosis helps differentiate between them, much overlap exists. Both DKA and HONK can be associated with lactic acidosis. Early diagnosis and treatment, guided by frequent biochemical monitoring, are critical to the successful management of these conditions.

## THE PATHOGENESIS OF HYPERGLYCAEMIC COMAS

### DIABETIC KETOACIDOSIS

Diabetic ketoacidosis is characterized by varying degrees of hyperglycaemia, raised blood ketone body concentrations and a metabolic acidosis. It occurs most frequently in patients with type 1 diabetes, but can occur under certain circumstances in those with type 2 diabetes. It can occur in individuals with established diabetes or can be the presenting feature. These metabolic abnormalities develop when there is a relative insulin deficiency in the presence of excess counter-regulatory hormones. Insulin deficiency is rarely absolute. In patients presenting with DKA, insulin concentrations are usually in the low physiological range, which would normally be sufficient to regulate lipolysis and hepatic glucose production. However, in the presence of elevated catabolic hormones, in particular glucagon and catecholamines (adrenaline and noradrenaline), resistance to the effects of insulin is seen. Conditions that result in excess circulating catabolic hormones include infections, trauma and myocardial infarction. Omission of insulin or reduction of dose, prompted by illness with or without inappropriate advice, often compounds the catabolic situation. In up to 40% of cases of DKA, no obvious precipitating cause is found.

Insulin promotes peripheral uptake and utilisation of glucose by skeletal muscle, adipose tissue and splanchnic tissues, and inhibits hepatic glucose production (from both glycogenolysis and gluconeogenesis) (*Figure 5.1*). Glucagon and catecholamines oppose these actions, reducing peripheral utilisation of glucose, promoting glycogen breakdown, and promoting gluconeogenesis from amino acids, lactate and glycerol (*Figure 5.2*). Gluconeogenesis in particular is enhanced, with an increased supply of amino acid precursors secondary to reduced protein synthesis and increased prote-olysis due to relative insulin deficiency. The resulting hyperglycaemia draws water from the intracellular to the extracellular compartment with an associated dilution of plasma sodium. Although the increase in plasma osmolality stimulates vasopressin secretion, its action is insufficient to compensate for the osmotic effect of glucose in the lumen of the nephrons and an osmotic diuresis results. Dehydration then leads to further release of counter-regulatory hormones and further exacerbates the insulin resistant state.

| Metabolic effects of insulin | | | | | |
|---|---|---|---|---|---|
| **Liver** | | **Muscle** | | **Adipocyte** | |
| Glycogenolysis | ↓↓↓ | Glucose uptake | ↑↑↑ | Glucose uptake | ↑↑↑ |
| Gluconeogenesis | ↓↓ | Ketone metabolism | ↑ | Lipolysis | ↓↓↓ |
| Ketogenesis | ↓ | | | | |

**Figure 5.1 Metabolic effects of insulin**

The elevation in blood ketone body concentrations (3-hydroxybutyrate and acetoac-etate, *Figure 5.3*) is driven by the high rates of lipolysis that occur in DKA. Catecholamines activate hormone-sensitive lipase, which mediates triglyceride breakdown to non-esterified fatty acids (NEFA) and glycerol. Insulin opposes this process, but in the presence of high catecholamine concentrations and a relative defi-ciency of insulin, lipolysis proceeds unchecked. The increased amounts of NEFA arriving at the liver are converted to coenzyme A derivatives and transported into the mitochondria (*Figure 5.3*). Within the mitochondria, partial oxidation of fatty acyl-coenzyme A (β-oxidation) leads to the formation of ketone bodies (*Figure 5.4*). Ketogenesis is further enhanced by decreased malonyl coenzyme A concentrations, which result from the increased ratio of glucagon to insulin in DKA. Malonyl coen-zyme A inhibits carnitine palmitoyl acyl transferase 1, the rate-limiting enzyme of ketogenesis. Ketone bodies are normally metabolized by conversion to acetyl CoA and subsequent oxidation, but this metabolic pathway is overwhelmed in DKA.

**Metabolic effects of catabolic hormones**

|  | Catecholamines | Glucagon | Cortisol | Growth hormone |
|---|---|---|---|---|
| **Liver** | | | | |
| Glycogenolysis | ↑↑↑ | ↑↑ | None | None |
| Gluconeogenesis | ↑ | ↑↑↑ | ↑↑↑ | ↑ |
| Ketogenesis | ↑ | ↑↑ | ↑ | ↑ |
| **Muscle** | | | | |
| Glucose uptake | ↓ | None | ↓↓ | ↓ |
| Ketone metabolism | ↓ | ? | ? | ? |
| **Adipocyte** | | | | |
| Glucose uptake | ↓ | None | ↓↓ | ↓ |
| Lipolysis | ↑↑↑ | None | ↑↑ | ↑ |

Key: ↑ = stimulatory, ↓ = inhibitory, none = no effect, ? = uncertain

Figure 5.2 Metabolic effects of catabolic hormones

**Ketone bodies**

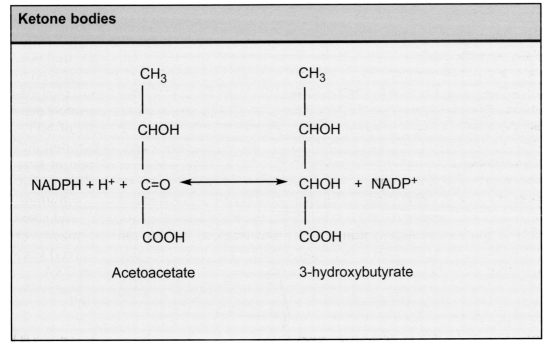

Figure 5.3 Ketone bodies

The acidosis that accompanies DKA is generated by the dissociation of ketone bodies (organic acids that dissociate fully at physiological $[H^+]$) to equimolar amounts of hydrogen ions and their respective anions. The body's buffering capacity (primarily bicarbonate) is soon exceeded, resulting in a metabolic acidosis with an increased anion gap $\{([Na^+] + [K^+]) - ([Cl^-] + [HCO_3^-])\}$. Acidosis itself further exacerbates insulin resistance. It also has a negative inotropic effect on cardiac muscle and causes peripheral vasodilatation, both of which contribute to systemic hypotension. The degrees of ketosis and acidosis are unrelated to the severity of the hyperglycaemia. Although most patients with DKA are hyperglycaemic, many cases of euglycaemic ketoacidosis have been described.

**Ketone body formation in the mitochondria**

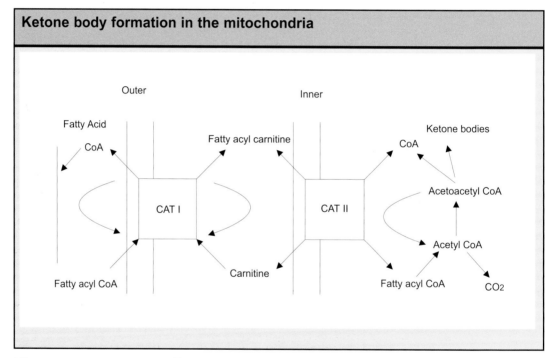

**Figure 5.4 Ketone body formation in the mitochondria**

A metabolic acidosis, also characterized by euglycaemia and ketonaemia, can occur in alcoholics. Following a drinking binge and vomiting, elevated concentrations of counter-regulatory hormones, due to dehydration and alcohol withdrawal, stimulate lipolysis and ketogenesis. In this situation, 3-hydroxybutyrate elevation is often much greater than that of acetoacetate, and nitroprusside-based ketone assays, which do not measure the former, may give misleading results.

Both hyperglycaemia and hyperketonaemia contribute to an osmotic diuresis, leading to dehydration and secondary losses of electrolytes (mainly sodium and potassium). Total body water deficit in DKA is often around 5-8 litres, whilst the sodium deficit can be 400-700 mmol. Although there is significant total body potassium depletion, patients are often hyperkalaemic because of the catabolic state and absolute or relative insulin deficiency, unless renal perfusion is well maintained. Plasma concentrations of potassium at presentation depend mainly on urinary losses. Magnesium and phosphate are also significantly depleted.

## HYPERGLYCAEMIC NON-KETOTIC COMA

Hyperglycaemic non-ketotic (HONK) coma is defined as the presence of hyperglycaemia (plasma glucose often above 50 mmol/L) without the marked hyperketonaemia and acidosis seen in DKA. One suggested working definition is plasma osmolality greater than 340 mmol/kg, less than 2+ ketonuria (Ketostix) and a plasma bicarbonate concentration greater than 18 mmol/L (unless lactic acidosis complicates the clinical picture). It usually occurs in older patients, in whom it may be the first presentation of type 2 diabetes, and also occurs more frequently in Afro-Caribbeans. Patients are often profoundly dehydrated and have a reduced level of consciousness. Mortality rates are around 30%, much higher than in patients with DKA, even with optimal management. This may reflect the high incidence of serious underlying disorders and complications found in this older age group.

The pathophysiology of HONK appears similar to that of DKA and indeed there is a degree of overlap between the two conditions. As in DKA, there is relative insulin deficiency in the presence of excess catabolic hormone concentrations. Precipitating factors are more commonly identified than in DKA. These include infections, myocardial infarction and stroke. The use of some drugs, particularly corticosteroids and thiazide diuretics, has also been implicated in the aetiology of HONK.

The hormonal changes that develop in patients with HONK cause uncontrolled output of glucose from the liver and some increase in lipolysis. However, it is unclear why the increased supply of NEFA to the liver does not lead to significant ketone body production in this condition. Plasma insulin concentrations are similar in HONK and DKA, so the argument that circulating insulin in HONK is just sufficient to hold lipolysis in check is not tenable. It is possible that the hyperosmolality found in HONK may have an inhibitory effect on lipolysis and ketogenesis.

Hyperglycaemia in patients with HONK is often severe. This reflects a longer presenting history during which time large amounts of glucose-containing drinks may have been consumed. Vomiting is uncommon, delaying the development of dehydration. Pre-existing renal disease, together with dehydration, can lead to a failure to excrete the glucose load and hence further accentuate the hyperglycaemia. In the absence of hyperketonaemia, significant acidosis does not occur, but may be found if lactic acidosis develops. The conditions precipitating HONK include infection and myocardial infarction, which can both be complicated by lactic acidosis. An acidosis may also develop secondarily to the prerenal renal failure that accompanies severe HONK.

LACTIC ACIDOSIS

Lactic acidosis occurs when the rates of production of lactate and hydrogen ions exceed those of their removal. Lactic acid is the product of anaerobic glycolysis, which occurs mainly in skeletal muscle, brain, erythrocytes and the renal medulla. Normally, lactate produced is converted to glucose and/or glycogen via gluconeogenesis in the liver and kidneys, or is oxidized to carbon dioxide and water (*see Figure 5.5*). Normal fasting blood lactate concentrations are 0.4 to 1.2 mmol/L. In clinically significant lactic acidosis, blood concentrations of lactate exceed 5 mmol/L with arterial $[H^+] > 45$ nmol/L (pH $< 7.35$).

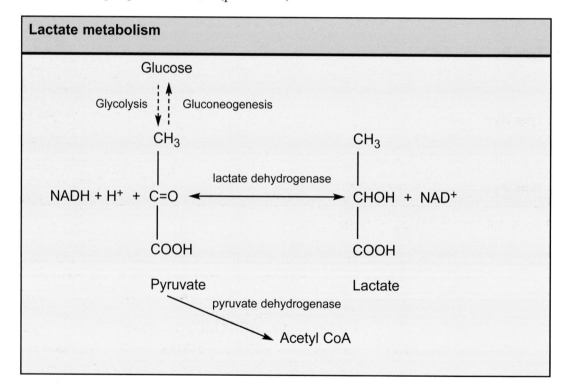

**Figure 5.5 Lactate metabolism**

Lactic acidosis can be congenital or acquired. Congenital forms of lactic acidosis are due to inborn errors of metabolism, which reflect genetic defects in gluconeogenesis, pyruvate dehydrogenase, the tricarboxylic acid cycle or the respiratory chain. These will not be discussed further. Acquired lactic acidosis may be classified into two general categories (*see Figure 5.6*). In type A lactic acidosis, tissue oxygen availability is inadequate to meet tissue demands (e.g. cardiogenic shock, asphyxia, carbon monoxide poisoning) and lactic acidosis is often a pre-terminal event. In type B, factors other than tissue hypoxia are the cause. Conditions where type B lactic acidosis occur include sepsis, liver failure, renal failure, diabetes and cancer. Several drugs and toxins can also be responsible. Most cases are mixtures of type A and type B and reflect problems in both the production and removal of lactate and hydrogen ions.

---

### Classification of lactic acidosis

| | |
|---|---|
| **Type A** | Associated with poor tissue perfusion |
| | Circulatory collapse |
| | Asphyxia |
| | Endotoxic shock |
| **Type B$_1$** | Associated with other diseases |
| | Hepatic disease |
| | Diabetes |
| **Type B$_2$** | Associated with drugs |
| | Biguanides |
| | Intravenous sorbitol, xylitol, fructose |
| **Type B$_3$** | Inborn errors of metabolism |

**Figure 5.6 Classification of lactic acidosis**

The prognosis of lactic acidosis is poor. Treatment of the underlying condition remains the mainstay of treatment. Intravenous bicarbonate has been, and continues to be, used extensively in severe lactic acidosis. However, no controlled trials have shown it to have any clinical efficacy. It appears that once arterial lactate concentration reaches 5 mmol/L, it is little more than a marker of the severity of the underlying illness and treating the acidosis *per se* does not have much value. Sodium dichloroacetate has also been used to treat lactic acidosis. It stimulates pyruvate dehydrogenase activity and hence lowers lactate concentrations, but has not been shown to reduce mortality.

Up to 10% of patients presenting with DKA have a raised plasma lactate concentration, which may contribute to their metabolic acidosis. An inhibitory effect of ketones on hepatic lactate uptake may in part be responsible. There may be a further transient rise in plasma lactate concentration when treatment of DKA is commenced. Insulin suppresses gluconeogenesis and hence hepatic lactate uptake, as well as promoting peripheral glucose uptake and utilisation, which generates more lactate.

Treatment of type 2 diabetes with biguanide drugs is associated with a risk of development of lactic acidosis. This was particularly the case with phenformin, which is no longer in use. However, it can occur, rarely, in patients treated with metformin, particularly in the presence of impaired renal function (a contraindication to the use of this drug). These drugs may favour conversion of glucose to lactate and can inhibit pyruvate oxidation to acetyl CoA. In the basal state, lactate concentrations in patients on these drugs are mildly elevated, but it is only in those in whom serious illnesses (e.g. renal failure, shock) intervene that lactic acidosis may develop.

## DIABETIC KETOACIDOSIS

### CLINICAL PRESENTATION
Most patients presenting with DKA complain of thirst and polyuria, which are secondary to the osmotic diuresis. Thirst is a result of the increased plasma osmolality, to which the diuresis contributes. Depending on the acuteness of the presentation, there may also be marked weight loss and fatigue. Nausea and vomiting are common and may aggravate the fluid and electrolyte loss. Abdominal pain can also occur and may be due to ketosis. If the pain does not settle within a few hours of treatment, other causes of abdominal pain should be sought, although it should be noted that plasma amylase activity is often increased in DKA, probably secondarily to reduced renal excretion, and does not signify pancreatitis.

At presentation, patients are usually dehydrated and hypotensive with a tachycardia. They also have the characteristic deep and rapid respiratory pattern (air hunger or Kussmaul breathing) that is seen with any metabolic acidosis. It can therefore also be present in those with lactic acidosis, but is not present in patients with HONK. The smell of ketones (like pear drops) may be detectable on the patient's breath, but many people are anosmic for this. Hypothermia may also be present and may be partly due to peripheral vasodilatation mediated by the acidosis. In severe cases of DKA, drowsiness leading to coma occurs but fewer than 25% of patients with DKA are comatose at presentation. The development of coma appears to correlate with plasma osmolality and plasma glucose concentration. It is thus more commonly seen in patients with HONK than in those with DKA. Intracellular fluid loss from cerebral cells may be a causal factor.

### LABORATORY FINDINGS AT PRESENTATION OF DKA
Diagnosis must be made as soon as possible so that appropriate therapy can be

commenced without delay. This should be possible in the casualty department based on the clinical presentation and bedside blood and urine tests. Capillary blood glucose concentration can be measured using a glucose meter, but the analytical range of meters is such that laboratory measurement is required to establish the severity of hyperglycaemia. Laboratory glucose analysis should continue to be used during treatment until concentrations fall to within the analytical range of the meter. Urine can be tested for glycosuria and for the presence of ketones using Ketostix dipsticks. Ketone detection by Ketostix is based on nitroprusside, which produces a purple colour on reaction with acetoacetate. However, in patients with DKA, acetoacetate concentrations are often considerably less than those of 3-hydroxybutyrate. These tests therefore provide a qualitative rather than a quantitative test for ketones. Arterial blood should be collected for measurement of hydrogen ion concentration or pH, $pCO_2$ and $pO_2$. Blood gas analysers automatically calculate 'standard bicarbonate' and base excess and most state-of-the-art systems include ion-selective electrodes for sodium and potassium, as well as for other analytes (e.g. glucose and lactate) in some cases. Patients with DKA have a metabolic acidosis with a raised hydrogen ion concentration (low pH) and low bicarbonate. The acidosis stimulates respiration and as respiratory compensation occurs, the $pCO_2$ will fall. Capillary blood can be used for [$H^+$] and $pCO_2$ measurement if it is impossible to obtain an arterial specimen. The $pO_2$ measurement is useful as hypoxia may cause a concomitant lactic acidosis. Other causes of a metabolic acidosis include chronic renal failure, alcoholic ketoacidosis and drug poisoning (e.g. with methanol, ethylene glycol, salicylates).

Venous blood should be taken for the measurement of glucose, urea, creatinine, sodium and potassium and a full blood count (neutrophilia is common in DKA and in itself does not indicate infection). Plasma sodium concentration is generally low at the start of treatment. This does not reflect the total body sodium deficit, but is due to the presence of hyperglycaemia, which draws water from the intracellular compartment, so diluting the plasma. An approximate correction for this phenomenon can be made by adding 1 mmol/L to the plasma sodium concentration for each 3 mmol/L elevation in plasma glucose. Raised plasma triglycerides may lead to falsely low sodium results (pseudohyponatraemia) if methods requiring specimen dilution, such as indirect ion selective electrode measurement, are used. This should be borne in mind when interpreting the rise in plasma sodium concentration that occurs during treatment as glucose and triglyceride concentrations fall.

Plasma potassium concentration is often raised at presentation despite the total body deficit of potassium. Metabolic acidosis promotes potassium efflux from cells in exchange for hydrogen ions, and renal hypoperfusion limits potassium loss. Other non-specific laboratory abnormalities seen in DKA include raised plasma activities of aminotransferases (transaminases) and creatine kinase, which may suggest a diagnosis of myocardial infarction. Absence of the ECG changes associated with infarction and the measurement of troponin I or troponin T should help rule this out. Elevated plasma amylase activity may suggest pancreatitis and abdominal pain may be present, adding further confusion.

## TREATMENT

### FLUID AND ELECTROLYTE REPLACEMENT

The essence of treatment of patients with DKA is rehydration and correction of electrolyte deficits, insulin administration to lower circulating glucose concentration, inhibit ketone body production and promote ketone clearance, and frequent clinical and laboratory monitoring.

Restoration of fluid and electrolyte deficits is the first priority. Isotonic saline (154 mmol/L; 0.9% saline) is usually given to restore plasma volume. Correction of plasma volume, even without insulin therapy, partly lowers plasma glucose, urea and potassium, although it does not affect the metabolic acidosis. Rehydration is also associated with a fall in the concentrations of counter-regulatory hormones, which helps to enhance the response to concurrent insulin treatment. Large amounts of fluid are required and most guidelines for fluid replacement aim at administering 5-8 litres of isotonic saline in the first 12-24 hours.

It is important that the plasma glucose concentration is carefully monitored during treatment and laboratory measurements should be used until the concentration falls to well within the measurement range of ward glucose meters. Once plasma glucose falls below 15 mmol/L, 5% or 10% glucose (dextrose) is given to allow the continued infusion of insulin required to control ketonaemia, whilst avoiding hypoglycaemia. Isotonic saline can be given concurrently if the patient is still dehydrated.

Special care may be needed with fluid replacement in older patients and in those with coexistent cardiovascular disease. Central venous pressure monitoring can be helpful in these situations. In those patients whose plasma sodium concentrations rise above 150 mmol/L during treatment, hypotonic saline (77 mmol/L; 0.45% saline) can be used. In children, there is some evidence that too rapid a correction of plasma glucose is associated with a higher risk of developing cerebral oedema. Subclinical brain swelling can be present at presentation of DKA, and may worsen with treatment. The development of clinically significant cerebral oedema may be associated with rapid rates of fluid replacement and glucose lowering.

Treatment of DKA with insulin and fluids corrects the acidosis and stimulates the movement of potassium from the extracellular to the intracellular compartment. Continuing renal loss of potassium, together with the shift of potassium into cells, can lead to hypokalaemia. This is potentially a life-threatening complication of the treatment of DKA and it is also entirely preventable if anticipated and monitored carefully. Potassium is not usually added to the first litre of saline infused, because the patient may be hyperkalaemic. However, once potassium concentrations are known, replacement therapy should be given if appropriate. If the potassium concentration is greater than 5.5 mmol/L, additional potassium can be omitted. At concentrations of potassium between 3.5 to 5.5 mmol/L, 20 mmol/L potassium chloride should be added to each litre of saline or dextrose. At potassium concentrations below 3.5 mmol/L, 40 mmol/L of potassium chloride should be added. It is essential to monitor potassium concentrations until the clinical and biochemical status of the patient has stabilized.

Phosphate is also depleted in patients with DKA, owing to urinary losses. During treatment, plasma phosphate concentration falls as phosphate enters cells. Plasma concentrations may fall into a range associated with impaired cardiac and skeletal muscle function, respiratory failure and rhabdomyolysis (< 0.3 mmol/L). However, these complications are rare. Hypophosphataemia can result in low erythrocyte 2,3-diphosphoglycerate (2,3-DPG) and impair tissue oxygenation. However, there is no evidence of clinical benefit when phosphate replacement is given during treatment of DKA.

*INSULIN ADMINISTRATION*

Insulin therapy is normally given by intravenous infusion pump, although it may be prudent to give a 10-20 unit bolus of intramuscular insulin immediately on diagnosis of DKA, while the infusion is prepared. This will serve to ensure continued insulin delivery if there are problems in obtaining venous access. Bolus intravenous administration of insulin is of limited use owing to its short half-life (approximately five minutes). Most guidelines suggest giving 6 units of short-acting insulin in solution in 0.9% saline/hour. This will result in plasma insulin concentrations around 100 mU/L. Insulin infusion should be continued at 6 units per hour until plasma glucose concentrations fall below 15 mmol/L: the rate can then be reduced to 3 units per hour, but insulin infusion should be continued until ketonaemia resolves. It is important to appreciate that an aim of insulin administration is to correct the metabolic acidosis. Indeed, this is more important than lowering plasma glucose concentrations. Correction of the acidosis will occur as ketone bodies are metabolised. In instances where plasma glucose declines satisfactorily during treatment but the acidosis persists uncorrected, it is inappropriate to reduce the infusion of insulin: insulin administration should be continued at the initial infusion rate or even doubled, and hypoglycaemia prevented by infusion of glucose. It follows, therefore, that there is no place for complex 'sliding scales' of insulin administration based on plasma glucose concentration in the management of DKA.

## BICARBONATE

The metabolic acidosis usually resolves with fluid and insulin replacement. It does not require specific therapy with alkali. Indeed, current evidence is that administration of sodium bicarbonate may be associated with adverse outcomes. Bicarbonate may exacerbate hypokalaemia, worsen intracellular acidosis owing to increased carbon dioxide production, and delay clearance of ketone bodies. There are two situations when bicarbonate might be considered: when [H$^+$] is greater than 110 nmol/L (pH < 6.9) and there is circulatory collapse, bicarbonate treatment may have a role to play, and when there is life-threatening hyperkalaemia at presentation. In these circumstances, 100 mmol of bicarbonate can be given. This should be given at the lowest concentration available for infusion, although few hospitals have anything other than 8.4% readily available. Because of the unpleasant side-effects of extravasation of this solution, 8.4% sodium bicarbonate must be given with care.

## OTHER CONSIDERATIONS

Attempts should be made to identify any precipitating causes of DKA, particularly infection or myocardial infarction. Quite how far a search for infection should proceed is unclear but it is sensible to examine an MSU and, if the patient is pyrexial, blood culture should be performed. The white cell count is of limited value in indicating infection in this condition as DKA is accompanied by a non-specific increase in circulating polymorphs.

Hypokalaemia and hypoglycaemia should be avoidable by judicious monitoring during treatment. Occasionally, however, other complications arise during treatment. The acute onset of breathlessness may herald the development of pulmonary oedema (or adult respiratory distress syndrome) while a catastrophic collapse usually suggests cerebral oedema.

Following correction of the metabolic abnormalities of DKA, stabilization of the patient and treatment of any precipitating medical cause, review of the ongoing treatment for his or her diabetes is essential. This should be done in liaison with the diabetes team in the hospital and the primary care team.

The published figures for mortality in this condition are of the order of 6%. Deaths occur mainly in the elderly or in patients in whom DKA is precipitated by a myocardial infarction: these patients are less able to absorb the fluid loads necessary for rehydration.

# HYPEROSMOLAR NON-KETOTIC HYPERGLYCAEMIA

## CLINICAL PRESENTATION

Patients with HONK often present with a depressed level of consciousness and there may be a history of up to three weeks of prior thirst, polyuria and increasing confusion. There is often a history of thirst quenching with drinks with a high sugar content. Vomiting and abdominal pain are not normally present. Severe dehydration and hypotension are much more frequent than in DKA. Focal neurological signs may occur but are normally reversible with treatment. However, venous and arterial thromboses also occur and may give rise to more permanent neurological deficits.

## LABORATORY FINDINGS

The diagnosis of HONK can be suggested by the clinical picture together with bedside monitoring. Significant ketosis and acidosis should be absent, although there may be a trace of ketones on urinalysis with Ketostix. In the presence of renal failure, shock or hypoxia, there may also be a lactic acidosis. Laboratory confirmation of the extent of elevation of plasma glucose and measurement of osmolality is required to confirm the diagnosis. HONK is characterized by fluid and electrolyte depletion, which can comprise as much as 25% of intra- and extra-cellular fluid. The osmotic diuresis leads to a hypotonic fluid loss. This effect, which raises plasma sodium concentration, can be masked by pseudohyponatraemia secondary to hypertriglyceridaemia. Thus plasma sodium concentration may be low, normal, or high. If sodium is normal or high despite these confounding factors, the water deficit is likely to be large.

Plasma osmolality can be measured in the laboratory using depression of freezing point or vapour pressure. Alternatively, osmolarity can be calculated using one of several published calculations. A widely used example is:

Plasma osmolarity (mmol/L) =

$$2 \times ([Na^+] + [K^+]) + [glucose] + [urea]$$

Results are often greater than 340 mmol/L in patients with HONK. In DKA, osmolality is increased, but is rarely greater than 320 mmol/L. Evidence of myocardial infarction as a precipitant must be sought. It should be noted that a raised plasma total creatine kinase activity may also be due to rhabdomyolysis, which can complicate HONK, and other cardiac markers, particularly the troponins, are likely to provide more information.

| Laboratory findings in DKA and HONK | | |
|---|---|---|
| Investigation | DKA | HONK |
| Plasma [glucose] | Raised to markedly high; occasionally normal | High to markedly high |
| Plasma [ketones] | High | Absent or low |
| Urine ketones | +++ | + to ++ |
| Plasma [sodium] | Low normal or raised | Raised |
| Plasma [potassium] | Low normal or raised | Raised |
| Plasma [bicarbonate] | Low | Normal |
| Blood [hydrogen ion] | High | Normal |
| Blood pH | Low | Normal |
| $PaCO_2$ | Low | Normal |
| Plasma osmolality | Raised | Markedly raised |

**Figure 5.7  Laboratory findings in DKA and HONK**

TREATMENT
Treatment of patients with HONK follows the same principles as those for the treatment of DKA. Underlying precipitants (infection, infarction, stroke) should be sought and treated appropriately. Fluid replacement needs to be more carefully managed and central venous access can be helpful to guide infusion rates. Plasma sodium frequently rises above 150 mmol/L and 0.45% saline is often required to limit this rise, although it is essential that rapid falls in plasma osmolality, which can cause rapid (and potentially harmful) shifts of water between the extra- and intracellular compartments, are avoided. Similar rates of insulin infusion and potassium replacement are used as in the treatment of DKA although potassium requirements are often less, as the patients are not acidotic. There appears to be a relatively high risk of thromboembolic disease in these patients and heparin may be given to try to prevent this complication.

Mortality rates in HONK approach 33%, probably reflecting the older age group of patients with this condition.

Patients who survive may not require long-term treatment with insulin although it is probably unwise to discontinue insulin too early. Oral agents or even diet alone may be sufficient treatment of the diabetes after the initial presentation.

## LACTIC ACIDOSIS

### CLINICAL PRESENTATION
Patients who present with lactic acidosis are usually ill from other major conditions. Type A lactic acidosis associated with hypoxia is the commonest presentation of this condition and may be difficult to diagnose clinically, as the patients are often already critically ill. The presentation may be put down solely to the presenting illness and the significance of the lactic acidosis be overlooked.

### LABORATORY FINDINGS
Lactic acidosis presents as a metabolic acidosis with circulating lactate concentrations > 5 mmol/L, without marked ketonaemia or ketonuria. It may be suspected if there is a raised anion gap and low bicarbonate in the absence of ketosis, although it is not uncommon to see minor degrees of ketosis. In many patients, neither the anion gap nor the hydrogen ion concentration is an accurate indication of the magnitude of the raised blood lactate. This is because raised lactate concentrations are also found in the presence of conditions such as liver failure and sepsis, which may themselves predispose to alkalosis. Respiratory alkalosis may also confuse the picture. Thus, laboratory measurement of lactate is required to confirm the diagnosis. The incorporation of ion selective electrodes for lactate into blood gas analysers has improved the availability of this analysis for acutely ill patients.

### TREATMENT
There are at least two occasions when lactic acidosis may be diagnosed yet no specific treatment is required. A metabolic acidosis with raised lactate concentration may be found after a grand mal fit. In the absence of other conditions, this is entirely self-correcting. Also, raised lactate in the presence of a metabolic acidosis may be found during treatment of DKA. Again, this requires no specific treatment in addition to that for DKA.

Currently, aggressive treatment of the underlying cause of the lactic acidosis remains the mainstay of therapy. A number of approaches to treatment have been tried but there is no convincing evidence of an alteration in outcome from these treatments from controlled trials. Large amounts of bicarbonate have been given (in excess of

3000 mmols) in an attempt to lower the hydrogen ion concentration on the basis that the liver becomes a lactate producer rather than a lactate user at an [H⁺] of approximately 80 nmol/L (pH 7.1). Such an approach demands extreme caution since it inevitably leads to a requirement for dialysis to remove the accompanying sodium ion. Insulin has also been used in an attempt to promote pyruvate metabolism but this will need accompanying glucose infusion. Again, this is not without danger since in the hypoxic state, insulin will promote glucose metabolism to lactate and exacerbate the situation. Experimental treatment has been tried with dichloroacetate, an activator of pyruvate dehydrogenase.

Mortality in patients with lactic acidosis is around 50% although given that the condition may be overlooked, the real figure may be higher than this.

## ROLE OF THE LABORATORY IN MONITORING THE RESPONSE TO TREATMENT

During the treatment of DKA and HONK, there are rapid changes in plasma glucose, sodium and potassium concentrations. Acid-base status must also be monitored, using either hydrogen ion concentration, which may be measured at the point of care, or less satisfactorily, plasma bicarbonate concentration. These must be closely monitored in order to prevent complications of therapy developing. In cases where plasma glucose is markedly raised (patients with HONK more so than those with DKA), bedside capillary glucose monitoring may be useless for several hours until glucose falls below around 30 mmol/L (i.e. within the range of handheld glucose meters). Laboratory glucose measurement is therefore essential to gauge the efficacy of treatment.

Assessment of ketonaemia is usually only done indirectly, by measurement of urinary ketones. As ketoacidosis improves with therapy, 3-hydroxybutyrate is converted to acetoacetate, sometimes resulting in a paradoxical increase in measured ketone bodies (acetoacetate). False positive tests with nitroprusside reagents have been reported to occur with sulphydryl drugs such as captopril, and exposure of the sample to air produces false negatives. Provided plasma bicarbonate is rising, Ketostix probably have little role in monitoring the response to treatment. Laboratory quantification of blood ketone bodies is seldom available. Recently, bedside blood ketone meters have been developed that measure 3-hydroxybutyrate. These may have some role both in initial diagnosis and in treatment. Normalisation of ketonaemia, as assessed by such monitoring, has been shown to require more prolonged treatment with high-dose insulin and dextrose. However, this has not been shown to influence clinical outcome.

Laboratory staff should be aware of the problems inherent in the measurement of plasma sodium concentrations in patients with DKA and HONK. Specimens must be directly observed to check for the presence of lipaemia. Flame emission and indirect ion selective electrode methods may give misleadingly low results in hyperlipidaemia (pseudohyponatraemia). Ideally, sodium concentrations in this situation are best measured using direct reading ion-selective electrodes and undiluted serum or whole blood. Knowledge of the clinical scenario and close liaison with the clinicians involved in the patient's care is important for a successful treatment outcome.

## FURTHER READING

Fulop M. Alcoholic ketoacidosis. Endocrin Metab Clin N America 1993; **22:** 209-19.

Krentz AJ, Nattrass M. Acute metabolic complications of diabetes mellitus: diabetic ketoacidosis, hyperosmolar non-ketotic syndrome and lactic acidosis. In: Pickup JC, Williams G, (eds). Textbook of Diabetes, (3rd edn). Oxford: Blackwell Science Ltd, 2003; pp 32.1-32.24.

Lebovitz HE. Diabetic ketoacidosis. Lancet 1995; **345:** 767-72.

Okuda Y, Adrogue HJ, Field JB *et al*. Counterproductive effects of sodium bicarbonate in diabetic ketoacidosis. J Clin Endocrin Metab 1996; **81:** 314-20.

Porter WH, Yao HH, Karounos DG. Laboratory and clinical evaluation of assays for β-hydroxybutyrate. Am J Clin Pathol 1997; **107:** 353-8.

Stacpoole PW. Lactic acidosis. Endocrin Metab Clin N America 1993; **22:** 221-45.

Umpierrez GE, Casals MMC, Gebhart SSP *et al*. Diabetic ketoacidosis in obese African-Americans. Diabetes 1995; **44:** 790-5.

Umpierrez GE, Watts NB, Phillips LS. Clinical utility of β-hydroxybutyrate determined by reflectance meter in the management of diabetic ketoacidosis. Diabetes Care 1995; **18:** 137-8.

Westphal SA. The occurrence of diabetic ketoacidosis in non-insulin-dependent diabetes and newly diagnosed diabetic adults. Am J Med 1996; **101:** 19-24.

Wiggam MI, O'Kane MJ, Harper R *et al*. Treatment of diabetic ketoacidosis using normalization of blood 3-hydroxybutyrate concentration as the endpoint of emergency management. Diabetes Care 1997; **20:** 1347-52.

# CLINICAL CASES

## DIABETIC KETOACIDOSIS

A 22 year old man, known to have type 1 diabetes, was admitted to hospital in a semi-comatosed state. Pulse rate 100/min, BP 105/70, respiratory rate 34/min.

Biochemistry results on admission:

| Analyte | Result | Reference range |
| --- | --- | --- |
| Sodium (mmol/L) | 130 | 134 -146 |
| Potassium (mmol/L) | 6.5 | 3.4 - 5.2 |
| Urea (mmol/L) | 32 | 3.4 - 8.0 |
| Creatinine (μmol/L) | 280 | 60 - 126 |
| Phosphate (mmol/L) | 1.2 | 0.8 - 1.4 |
| Glucose (mmol/L) | 59 | |
| **Arterial blood gases** | | |
| $[H^+]$ (nmol/L) | 60 | 35 - 45 |
| $pCO_2$ (kPa) | 2.8 | 4.7 - 6.0 |
| $pO_2$ (kPa) | 14 | 10 - 14 |
| $[HCO_3^-]$ (mmol/L) | 12 | 22 - 26 |
| **Urinalysis** | | |
| | Glucose ++++ | |
| | Protein 0 | |
| | Ketones ++ | |

Treatment was with intravenous 'normal' saline (154 mmol/L) and insulin infusion. After three hours, potassium chloride was added to the infusion.

| Time (hours) | 3 | 6 | 12 | 18 |
|---|---|---|---|---|
| Sodium (mmol/L) | 136 | 138 | 140 | 138 |
| Potassium (mmol/L) | 3.0 | 3.8 | 4.0 | 3.9 |
| Urea (mmol/L) | 18 | 14 | 9 | 8 |
| Creatinine (μmol/L) | 160 | 120 | 105 | 85 |
| Phosphate (mmol/L) | 1.02 | 0.76 | 0.70 | 0.67 |
| Plasma glucose (mmol/L) | 31 | 15 | 12 | 7 |
| $HCO_3^-$ (mmol/L) | 18 | 20 | 23 | 24 |
| Arterial [$H^+$] (nmol/L) | 52 | 47 | 42 | 40 |

The patient made a full recovery.

*POINTS*

1) Typical initial biochemical features of a diabetic ketoacidosis are:

- hyperglycaemia

- metabolic acidosis

- raised plasma and urine ketones

- hyperkalaemia

- raised plasma creatinine and urea (due to dehydration – the disproportionate increase is urea compared to creatinine is typical of dehydration and is exacerbated in DKA by urea production from amino acid breakdown)

- hypophosphataemia, which becomes more marked during treatment owing to cellular uptake of phosphate.

2. Treatment is with rehydration and infusion of insulin.

3. The principal aim of treatment is to correct the acidosis (this is more important in terms of morbidity and mortality than correcting the hyperglycaemia).

4. Insulin therapy promotes an intracellular shift of potassium. Therefore, serum potassium concentrations need to be closely monitored and potassium replacement is often required. (Most patients presenting with DKA are both sodium and potassium depleted despite being hyperkalaemic.)

5. The Ketostix method for ketone detection may give false negative results for ketonuria. This is because the basis of the method is the nitroprusside test, in which reaction occurs with acetoacetate but not β-hydroxybutyrate. In the early stages of DKA, the β-hydroxybutyrate:acetoacetate ratio is 8:1 owing to the large amounts of NADH, which favours β-hydroxybutyrate production. With appropriate treatment of the DKA, β-hydroxybutyrate is converted to acetoacetate and the Ketostix reaction becomes more positive.

6. Infusion of sodium bicarbonate is rarely necessary in DKA but may be used if there is severe acidosis leading to respiratory depression. When used, it should be given with extreme caution. Excretion of potassium is enhanced and this may lead to sudden hypokalaemia. Intramitochondrial oxidation of ketone bodies generates alkali: this is the most appropriate way to correct the acidosis.

7. The Jaffe reaction for creatinine measurement is subject to positive interference by high acetoacetate concentrations: this can occasionally result in artefactually raised creatinine concentrations.

## HYPEROSMOLAR NON-KETOTIC DIABETIC COMA (HONK)

A 61 year old women was admitted to hospital via her family doctor. She had complained of a flu-like illness for four days with a cough productive of yellow-green phlegm, for which she had been commenced on antibiotics (Augmentin®). For two days prior to admission she had complained of excessive thirst and polyuria. She had been quenching her thirst with fruit squash and Lucozade®. There was no prior history of diabetes. That morning she had been found in a semi-comatose state by her daughter.

On examination she was drowsy and clinically dehydrated.

Biochemistry results on admission:

| Analyte | Result | Reference range |
| --- | --- | --- |
| Sodium (mmol/L) | 158 | 134 -146 |
| Potassium (mmol/L) | 5.0 | 3.4 - 5.2 |
| Urea (mmol/L) | 32.7 | 3.4 - 8.0 |
| Creatinine (µmol/L) | 293 | 60 - 126 |
| Total protein (g/L) | 90 | 60 - 80 |
| Osmolality (mmol/kg) | 440 | 278 - 294 |
| Plasma glucose (mmol/L) | 83 | |
| **Arterial blood gases** | | |
| $[H^+]$ (nmol/L) | 44 | 35 - 45 |
| $pCO_2$ (kPa) | 6.0 | 4.7 - 6.0 |
| $pO_2$ (kPa) | 12 | 10 - 14 |
| $[HCO_3^-]$ (mmol/L) | 24 | 22 - 26 |
| **Urinalysis** | | |
| Glucose ++++ Ketones 0 | | |

A diagnosis of hyperosmolar non-ketotic diabetic coma was made.

Treatment was with intravenous 'normal' saline and insulin. The patient was also heparinised.

| Time (hours) | 6 | 18 |
|---|---|---|
| Sodium (mmol/L) | 166 | 144 |
| Potassium (mmol/L) | 4.5 | 4.2 |
| Urea (mmol/L) | 29.5 | 12 |
| Creatinine (μmol/L) | 240 | 150 |
| Plasma glucose (mmol/L) | 50 | 12 |

*POINTS:*

1. Hyperosmolar non-ketotic diabetic coma may be the presenting feature of type 2 diabetes.

2. Precipitating factors include infection, myocardial infarction and drugs (e.g. diuretics, steroids, antibiotics).

3. Initial biochemistry confirms dehydration, hyperglycaemia (plasma glucose often > 50 mmol/L and sometimes up to 100 mmol/L), hyperosmolar plasma but the absence of ketones or metabolic acidosis.

4. In the early stages of treatment, plasma sodium concentration rises owing to cellular uptake of glucose and water from the ECF. It may be necessary to switch from isotonic fluids for rehydration (0.9%, 154 mmol/L, 'normal' saline) to hypotonic saline (75 mmol/L). Infusion of hypotonic fluid is not without risk and a maximum of two litres should be given.

5. Heparin is sometimes given as anti-thrombosis prophylaxis in view of blood hyperviscosity.

# Chapter 6

# The biochemistry of diabetic complications

## INTRODUCTION

The discovery of insulin in 1922 changed type 1 diabetes from being a disease that was usually fatal within months of onset to one for which long term survival was theoretically possible. With this, however, came a new problem – the appearance of the long-term complications of the disease, many of which were already seen in the more common type 2 diabetes. These complications fall broadly into the microvascular complications, that is, retinopathy, nephropathy and, in part, neuropathy, and the macrovascular complications from accelerated atheroma formation throughout the arterial tree.

The complications of diabetes have serious consequences for both patients and health services. In the UK, diabetes is the commonest cause of blindness in people of working age, the most common indication for renal dialysis and transplantation, and second only to trauma as a reason for leg amputations. Most patients with diabetes die of cardiovascular disease and their mortality from myocardial infarction is twice that of the non-diabetic population. On average, diabetes reduces a person's life expectancy by one third from the time of diagnosis.

## THE PATHOGENESIS OF MICROANGIOPATHY

The development of the microvascular (or microangiopathic) complications of diabetes is associated with chronic hyperglycaemia: good glycaemic control modifies both their development and progression. Hyperglycaemia produces both acute, reversible, and chronic, irreversible, metabolic changes. Acutely, hyperglycaemia induces the intracellular accumulation of sorbitol via the polyol pathway, competes with myoinositol for cellular uptake, inhibits $Na^+$, $K^+$-ATPase leading to intracellular sodium accumulation and alters the cellular redox potential. Chronically, glycation of long-lived proteins leads to basement membrane changes, changes in the expression of genes, reduced blood vessel dilatation and enhanced atheroma formation.

## SORBITOL AND THE POLYOL PATHWAY (*Figure 6.1*)

The cellular uptake of glucose that is not mediated by insulin is dependent on the glucose concentration gradient across the cell membrane. In the presence of normoglycaemia, intracellular glucose is metabolised via the glycolytic pathway. A second pathway, the polyol pathway, in which glucose is reduced to sorbitol, its sugar alcohol, by aldose reductase and nicotinic acid dinucleotide phosphate (NADPH), is only a minor pathway because of the high Km of the enzyme. In the presence of hyperglycaemia, this pathway becomes much more important and intracellular concentrations of sorbitol rise owing to greater flux along the pathway and poor clearance of sorbitol, which does not diffuse easily across cell membranes. Sorbitol increases the osmotic pressure within cells and causes them to swell. This occurs during the formation of diabetic cataracts.

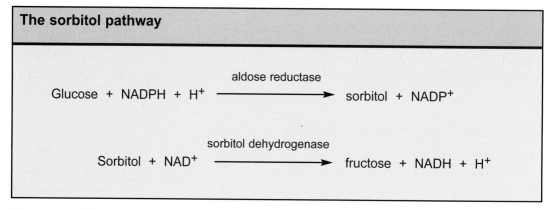

Figure 6.1 The sorbitol pathway

Sorbitol is then oxidised to fructose by sorbitol dehydrogenase and $NAD^+$. Consequently, the intracellular $NADH/NAD^+$ ratio rises and the redox potential is altered. This may affect DNA repair, fatty acid oxidation and promote the formation of diacylglycerol (DAG).

In the glycolytic pathway, the conversion of glyceraldehyde 3-phosphate to 1,3- diphosphoglycerate relies on the reduction of $NAD^+$ to NADH, which is slowed by an increase in the $NADH/NAD^+$ ratio. An alternative fate for glyceraldehyde 3-phosphate is metabolism by the diacylglycerol phosphate pathway to dihydroxy-acetone phosphate, which is itself reduced to glycerol 3-phosphate by the oxidation of NADH to $NAD^+$. This pathway ends with the formation of diacylglycerol, which binds to and activates protein kinase C. Protein kinase C increases vascular permeability, alters vascular blood flow and stimulates basement membrane synthesis, all of which are linked to the development of diabetic complications.

MYOINOSITOL AND $Na^+$, $K^+$-ATPase

In certain cells, accumulation of sorbitol is associated with depletion of alternative organic intracellular physiological osmolytes such as myoinositol. Myoinositol is a sugar alcohol with similarities to glucose. The main source is the diet, although it can be synthesized from glucose 6-phosphate. It competes with glucose for uptake into insulin independent tissues and its uptake is reduced in the presence of hypergly-caemia. People with diabetes are reported to have lower intracellular concentrations of myoinositol than those without but this is not a consistent finding. Intracellular myoinositol is converted to phosphoinositides. These mobilise calcium, which, with DAG, activates protein kinase C, which in turn activates $Na^+,K^+$-ATPase. $Na^+,K^+$-ATPase activity is reduced in insulin independent tissues in patients with diabetes. This causes an increase in the intracellular sodium concentration, which alters trans-membrane potentials and cellular function. As a result, nerve conduction velocity is reduced in patients with diabetes. Dietary myoinositol supplements and aldose reductase inhibitors (which, by reducing sorbitol formation, reduce the intracellular depletion of myoinositol) increase nerve conduction velocities but do not protect the kidney or retina from damage: no trials have shown an improved clinical outcome with these agents.

PROTEIN GLYCATION
Amino groups in proteins undergo non-enzymatic glycation in the presence of hyperglycaemia. The extent of this reaction depends on the degree and duration of the hyperglycaemia. Initially, a Schiff base is formed but this is stabilized by rearrangement, to form an Amadori product (*Figure 6.2*).

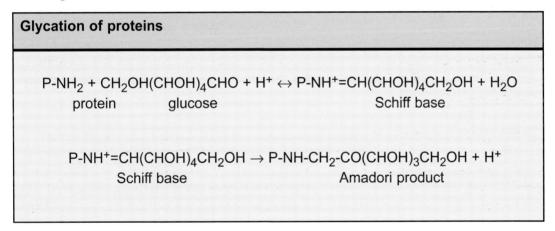

**Glycation of proteins**

$$P-NH_2 + CH_2OH(CHOH)_4CHO + H^+ \leftrightarrow P-NH^+=CH(CHOH)_4CH_2OH + H_2O$$

protein      glucose             Schiff base

$$P-NH^+=CH(CHOH)_4CH_2OH \rightarrow P-NH-CH_2-CO(CHOH)_3CH_2OH + H^+$$

Schiff base            Amadori product

**Figure 6.2 Glycation of proteins**

Amadori products are formed irreversibly and survive for the lifespan of the protein. Some proteins, such as collagen, are long lived and the Amadori products can undergo further, irreversible transformation to produce advanced glycation end-products (AGE). These form either by the condensation of two Amadori products or the reaction of an Amadori product with sugar fragments to form a pyrrole ring, which then reacts with the amino groups on other proteins. Both routes lead to the cross-linking of proteins, and hence alteration in their structure and, potentially, their function.

# ADVANCED GLYCATION END-PRODUCTS

## *BASEMENT MEMBRANE EFFECTS*

Circulating proteins such as albumin and immunoglobulins bind to the matrix of basement membranes covalently and undergo glycation. This binding increases the lifespan of the proteins, which would otherwise be cleared from the circulation, and increases the thickness and structure of the basement membrane. The membrane structure is also changed by the crosslinking between collagen and other proteins of the basement membrane that occurs when they are glycated. Structural and electrostatic changes consequent on this alter the thickness and function of basement membranes in the microcirculation. There is also loss of the normal regulation of basement membrane formation and an increase in extracellular matrix formation. These structural and functional changes are seen in diabetic nephropathy as an increase in extracellular deposits within the glomeruli and leakage of protein through the basement membrane.

## *INTRACELLULAR EFFECTS*

Within the cell, several sugars can form AGE with intracellular proteins. These sugars can also react with the primary amino groups of DNA nucleotides to form AGE. *In vitro* these have been associated with increased DNA breaks, repair and altered gene expression. AGE modification of gene expression or of intracellular proteins may alter cell function and thus, for example, vascular or neuronal function.

## *AGE RECEPTORS*

Receptors for AGE proteins are present on the surface of macrophages and endothelial cells. These receptors have a protein unit within the membrane, which has homology with immunoglobulin receptors. Stimulation of these receptors in endothelial cells leads to the intracellular production of oxygen free radicals and the activation of genes associated with an injury response. In macrophages, they induce the local production of monokines such as insulin-like growth factor 1 (IGF-1), interleukin 1 (IL-1) and tumour necrosis factor alpha (TNF-$\alpha$), which, in the kidney, stimulate the proliferation of glomerular mesangial cells, the glomerular production of type IV collagen (which is found in basement membranes) and the proliferation of arterial smooth muscle cells.

At the endothelium, activated AGE receptors also inhibit the activation of the anti-coagulant protein kinase C pathway, stimulate coagulant activity through factors IX and X and stimulate the production of endothelin-1, a vasoconstrictor. This leads to an increase in local thrombogenesis and vasoconstriction.

## SCREENING AND MONITORING OF MICROALBUMINURIA

Our understanding of the natural history of diabetic nephropathy and the value of screening for, and treating it, comes largely from two large randomised controlled trials in diabetes, the Diabetes Control and Complications Trial (DCCT) and United Kingdom Prospective Diabetes Study (UKPDS), in type 1 and type 2 diabetes, respectively.

In type 1 diabetes, the development of microalbuminuria is the earliest clinically detectable stage of the development of diabetic nephropathy. Microalbuminuria is not seen before the onset of puberty and rarely occurs within the first five years of diagnosis. Microalbuminuria may be a transient state that reverts to normal, remains stable or progresses to frank proteinuria. Once frank proteinuria has developed, the median survival is ten years. Only 35-40% of type 1 diabetic patients will develop diabetic nephropathy with most developing it within 15-20 years of diagnosis of diabetes but once diabetic nephropathy develops, it progresses inexorably to end stage renal failure.

Microalbuminuria is a urinary albumin excretion above the 95th centile of a non-diabetic population but which is not detectable with standard dipsticks (e.g. Albustix®). This is commonly taken to be a urinary albumin excretion rate of 20-200 µg/min (30-300 mg/24h). Because of a lack of prospective data, this range does not have any predictive value about the likelihood of progression to frank proteinuria or the value of any intervention; microalbuminuria itself may be increased by exercise, urinary tract infections, acute illness, cardiac failure or hypertension.

The detection of microalbuminuria requires the use of a sensitive albumin method and immunologically based systems, usually immunoturbimetry, are generally used. There are several ways of expressing the results. Twenty-four hour excretion or the excretion in a timed urine sample can be used but these are vulnerable to patient error and may be inconvenient. It is difficult to use these for screening. A spot urine albumin concentration can be measured either in the laboratory or with Micral® sticks, but can be affected by a patient's state of hydration and the timing of the sample: urinary albumin excretion is reduced by 30-50% overnight. This can be corrected for by measuring an albumin/creatinine (A/C) ratio. An A/C ratio > 2.5 mg/mmol in men or 3.5 mg/mmol in women (who have a lower creatinine excretion than men) suggests microalbuminuria.

Because of the variation in urine albumin excretion, the test should be positive on two out of three occasions over 3-6 months to confirm microalbuminuria. Once microalbuminuria has been confirmed, a timed collection can be done to quantify the excretion. Either A/C ratios or periodic timed urine collections can be used for follow up. Measurement of serum creatinine or creatinine clearance is not of use in diabetic nephropathy before the development of persistent clinical (Albustix positive) proteinuria.

Screening for microalbuminuria in post-pubertal type 1 patients should start five years after diagnosis and be performed annually for at least 20 years, after which the number of new cases would be expected to be few. People with type 1 diabetes can have non-diabetic causes of nephropathy and those screening for diabetic nephropathy should be alert for atypical cases of proteinuria in diabetic patients, e.g. proteinuria too early in the disease or proteinuria in the absence of diabetic retinopathy. In type 2 diabetes, there is no evidence from clinical trials to recommend a screening policy. In young type 2 patients, some would extrapolate and apply data from trials in type 1 diabetes, but in the older population this would be difficult to justify because non-diabetic causes of proteinuria, such as cardiac failure, and non-diabetic causes of nephropathy, such as ischaemia and atheromatous renal artery stenosis, occur more frequently.

## PATHOPHYSIOLOGY OF DYSLIPIDAEMIA

The dyslipidaemia of diabetes mellitus is characterised by raised serum triglyceride and very low-density lipoprotein (VLDL) concentrations, a low high-density lipoprotein cholesterol (HDL-C) concentration and a preponderance of small triglyceride-rich low-density lipoprotein (LDL) and HDL particles. Diabetes mellitus is itself a predisposing factor to macrovascular disease and the co-existence of abnormal lipid biochemistry increases cardiac risk. Good glycaemic control in type 1 diabetes mellitus is associated with normal plasma lipid concentrations and HDL may even become elevated, but in the insulin resistant state of type 2 diabetes, an abnormal lipid profile may persist despite good glycaemic control.

### GLYCATION OF APOLIPOPROTEINS

One factor common to all classes of lipoproteins in diabetes is that the apolipoprotein components of the lipid complexes are susceptible to increased glycation, as are all plasma proteins, because of the elevated prevailing glucose concentration. This glycation is thought to delay clearance of lipoprotein particles, probably by affecting binding at receptor sites.

### CHYLOMICRONS, VLDL AND TRIGLYCERIDE METABOLISM

The raised triglycerides in diabetes mellitus are primarily due to the altered modulation of the activities of lipoprotein lipase and hormone-sensitive lipase by insulin. Lipoprotein lipase activity is located on the endothelial surfaces of blood vessels in peripheral tissues, most importantly adipose tissue and muscle cells. It acts on both chylomicrons and VLDL, hydrolysing triglycerides and releasing free fatty acids, which are either metabolised as an energy source or, in adipocytes, are re-esterified with α-glycerophosphate to form storage triglyceride. The activity of lipoprotein lipase is increased by insulin, so in the actual or relative insulin deficient state prevailing in diabetes mellitus, there is reduced removal of triglycerides from chylomicron and VLDL particles, leading to high plasma concentrations of triglyceride, chylomicrons and large, triglyceride-rich VLDL particles. In the uncontrolled diabetic state, chylomicron clearance is markedly impaired, leading to visible lipaemia in the plasma. Institution of insulin treatment rapidly corrects this.

Hormone-sensitive lipase acts in adipose tissue to break down stored triglycerides and thus mobilises fat stores for utilisation. For metabolic efficiency, the enzyme activity is required to be greatest in the fasting state and suppressed on feeding; this is mediated by insulin, which inhibits hormone-sensitive lipase. In diabetes mellitus, this inhibition is lost or reduced and breakdown of stored fat continues, even in the fed state. This leads to uncontrolled release of free fatty acids into the circulation and their increased, concentration-dependent uptake by the liver.

Although some free fatty acids are metabolised via β-oxidation, in situations of excess, re-esterification with glycerol to form triglyceride and subsequent VLDL synthesis and release will be enhanced. Because of the increased availability of substrate in the insulin deficient state, not only is VLDL production increased, but the lipoproteins produced are rich in triglyceride, compounding the effects of insulin deficiency on the activity of lipoprotein lipase.

HDL AND LDL METABOLISM
The metabolism of the major cholesterol-transporting lipoproteins, HDL and LDL, is also altered significantly in diabetes mellitus.

*High density lipoprotein (HDL)*
HDL has a protective function with respect to cardiovascular disease in that it incorporates free cholesterol from peripheral tissues and facilitates its transport to the liver for disposal. It also acts as an antioxidant, limiting the lipid peroxidation that encourages atheroma formation. When HDL metabolism is disturbed, as in diabetes, its protective functions are reduced.

In normal circumstances, nascent HDL particles released from the liver become progressively less dense as they acquire apolipoproteins A and C (apoA and apoC) from other lipoproteins and free cholesterol from lipoproteins and cell membranes. Lecithin cholesterol acyl transferase (LCAT) converts the cholesterol to cholesteryl esters, which are incorporated into the HDL core, increasing the particle volume and surface area so that more apolipoproteins, phospholipid and free cholesterol can be accepted into the surface layers.

HDL particles are subdivided into two populations, based on their size. Nascent HDL and the smaller particles are classed as $HDL_3$. The larger particles, which have acquired more cholesterol, phospholipids and apolipoproteins, are termed $HDL_2$. In diabetes, where VLDL and chylomicron metabolism is disturbed as described above, there is reduced transfer of apolipoproteins and phospholipid to the surface of HDL, resulting in a preponderance of small, dense, $HDL_3$ particles and a low circulating HDL cholesterol concentration.

$HDL_2$ particles play a major role in the transfer of cholesterol to the liver for excretion or utilisation in synthetic processes. This is effected by the transfer of cholesteryl ester from $HDL_2$ to VLDL, chylomicrons and their remnant particles. These lipoproteins either undergo receptor-mediated uptake by the liver or, in the case of intermediate density lipoprotein (IDL), the remnant particle of VLDL, are converted to LDL.

The transfer of cholesteryl esters from $HDL_2$ is mediated by the action of cholesteryl ester transfer protein (CETP). In diabetes, there is excessive transfer of triglyceride to $HDL_2$ from remnant particles during this process, leading to triglyceride-enrichment of HDL particles.

*LOW DENSITY LIPOPROTEIN*
Most LDL is produced from IDL, although a small amount is synthesised in the liver. LDL is taken up by liver and peripheral cells by two different mechanisms, one mediated by the LDL receptor, the other following degradation of oxidised LDL by macrophages. The macrophages are converted to foam cells, the building blocks of atheromatous plaques, as they accumulate cholesteryl esters. LDL is therefore a major factor in the pathogenesis of cardiovascular disease and atherosclerosis. In DM, the altered transfer of lipid and protein components between the lipoproteins leads to the production of a population of small, dense LDL particles, which are preferentially cleared via the macrophage route, unlike larger, buoyant particles. There are two reasons for this. First, glycation of apoB, the apolipoprotein of LDL, reduces the affinity of the lipoprotein for the LDL receptor, thus reducing clearance by that mechanism. Second, these smaller particles are more susceptible to oxidation by free radicals and subsequent degradation by macrophages, thus increasing foam cell formation and the potential for the development of atheroma. Oxidised LDL may also be directly toxic to endothelial cells. Free radical activity is increased, and vitamin E and ascorbate concentrations decreased, in DM, creating ideal conditions for peroxidation of lipoproteins to occur and for the process leading to atheroma formation to be triggered. The presence of small, dense LDL particles has been shown to be powerfully and independently predictive of coronary events and the development of atherosclerotic disease.

It should be remembered that primary hyperlipidaemias are not uncommon disorders and occur in DM with the same frequency as in the non-diabetic population. The risk of cardiovascular disease is even higher in patients in whom DM and a primary lipid disorder coexist.

## EVIDENCE FOR TREATMENT OF HYPERLIPIDAEMIA IN DIABETES

Most people with diabetes die cardiovascular deaths and all are subject to the same risk factors for coronary heart disease that apply to the general population. The decision to screen for and treat hyperlipidaemia should be taken as part of a more general consideration of the individual's cardiovascular risk factors, i.e. lack of exercise, overweight, smoking, hypertension, family history, etc. Until recently, there had been no trials of lipid lowering therapy specifically in diabetes in which total or cardiovascular mortality had been a trial endpoint. Evidence for treatment had to be taken from trials in populations without diabetes or from trials in which subjects with diabetes were included. Nevertheless, there was evidence of benefit from lipid lowering in both primary (no previous history of CHD) and secondary (pre-existing CHD) trials, and patients with diabetes are at generally increased risk of CHD whatever their lipid status. Therefore, many physicians have been accustomed to treat these patients as if they were candidates for primary prevention and have had a low threshold for intervention with lipid lowering drugs if patients do not achieve a plasma cholesterol concentration < 5.0 mmol/L (LDL < 3.0) with dietary and lifestyle intervention alone.

Of particular importance in this respect were the Scandinavian Simvastatin Survival Study (4S) and the Cholesterol and Recurrent Events (CARE) trials, both trials of secondary prevention.

4S was a study of 4,444 men and women with angina or a previous myocardial infarction (MI), a cholesterol of 5.5-8.0 mmol/L and triglycerides < 2.3 mmol/L, who were treated with either placebo or simvastatin 20-40 mg o.d., and followed up for five years. There was a significant reduction in all cause mortality with simvastatin (256 (12%) deaths *vs* 182 (8%)). The cardiac mortality was reduced by 42% (189 (8.5%) placebo deaths *vs* 111 (5%) simvastatin). In the 202 subjects with diabetes there was no significant reduction in overall coronary mortality (17 *vs* 12 deaths) but there was a significant 50% reduction in all major coronary events (44 (45.4%) *vs* 24 (22.9%)).

The CARE trial, of pravastatin, studied 4,159 men and post-menopausal women who had had an MI and had a cholesterol of < 6.2 mmol/L and triglycerides < 4 mmol/L. The median follow up was five years. In the pravastatin treated group overall, there was a 24% reduction in fatal coronary events or non-fatal MIs (274 (13.2%) vs 212 (10.3%)), and in the 586 subjects with diabetes the reduction was also significant at 25% (112 (37%) vs 81 (29%)).

These trials illustrate the increased mortality of people with diabetes who have coronary artery disease or who have had an MI. The CARE trial also showed the benefit of treating a more diabetic lipid profile. On the basis of these studies it was recommended that patients with diabetes and angina or a history of MI should have their lipids measured and treatment with a statin should be started if the cholesterol was > 5.0 mmol/L, provided that they did not have markedly raised TGs, when a fibrate might be preferred. The benefits of fibrate treatment have also been demonstrated in large trials, e.g. the Helsinki Heart Study, albeit this included few patients with DM.

In the Helsinki Heart Study, a primary prevention trial, it was demonstrated that treatment with gemfibrozil (a fibrate-type drug) reduced myocardial infarction and cardiac death in middle-aged men with a non-HDL cholesterol > 5.2 mmol/L. There was a significant 34% reduction in cardiac deaths and events but no reduction in overall mortality in the treatment group. There were too few subjects with diabetes in the trial to draw any conclusions about them. The West of Scotland Coronary Prevention Study (WOSCOPS) (also a primary prevention trial) showed a reduction in cardiac events using pravastatin but there is no separate information available on diabetic patients.

However, the benefits of statin treatment in patients with diabetes were clearly demonstrated in the Heart Protection Study, published in 2003. This study involved 5,923 patients with diabetes aged between 40 and 80. Treatment with simvastatin 40 mg daily resulted in a reduction of vascular events (major coronary events, strokes and revascularisation procedures) of 22% over a five year period in comparison with controls. In subjects with no evidence of vascular disease on entry to the trial, the reduction was 33% and, of particular significance, a reduction of 27% was seen in patients with diabetes whose LDL cholesterol concentrations were < 3.0 mmol/L on entry to the trial.

The authors recommended that treatment with simvastatin 40 mg be considered for all patients with diabetes who are at high risk of vascular disease, irrespective of their LDL cholesterol concentrations. Current recommendations for intervention on the basis of cholesterol measurements are for target values of < 4.5 mmol/L for total cholesterol and < 2.5 mmol/L for LDL cholesterol.

## INFECTIONS AND DIABETES

The early literature in diabetes reported an excess mortality from infections. This is no longer the case but there are a few, rare, infective conditions that are peculiar to diabetes (mucormycosis, malignant otitis externa, emphysematous pyelonephritis and emphysematous cholecystitis). Generally, people with diabetes are susceptible to the same infections as others although their polymorphonuclear leucocyte (PMN) function is altered by hyperglycaemia and acidosis. The response to infection in diabetes is complex and incompletely understood.

Early work on PMNs in diabetes demonstrated a delayed early migration of neutrophils to a site of infection but after 24 hours their response was the same as in non-diabetics. This response was further reduced by acidosis but was unaffected by the prevailing glucose concentration and could be improved by insulin. Later work has shown a reduced PMN adherence to vascular endothelium *in vitro*.

*In vitro* studies of PMN phagocytosis of bacteria have shown that this is impaired in the presence of acidosis but the effects of hyperglycaemia have been variable. The serum of diabetic patients can impair the phagocytic activity of PMNs from subjects who do not have the disease. This suggests that there is an opsonization defect in the diabetic response to infection.

Hyperglycaemia reduces the bactericidal activity of PMNs. Stimulated PMNs require free radicals and hydrogen peroxide, which they produce in bursts of oxidative metabolism, to kill phagocytosed bacteria. Hyperglycaemia activates the sorbitol pathway with the consumption of NADPH. A fall in the intracellular NADPH concentration reduces PMN superoxide production, which is NADPH dependent, and thus its bactericidal activity and its ability to increase bactericidal activity in the presence of infection.

Infection is a frequent precipitant of hyperglycaemia in patients with diabetes, and specifically of ketoacidosis in type 1 DM. It should always be considered in the investigation and treatment of these patients. The stress of infection increases the secretion of hormones antagonistic to insulin (glucagon, growth hormone, cortisol and catecholamines). The resulting hyperglycaemia will impair bactericidal activity and acidosis will impair PMN migration and phagocytosis. Thus hyperglycaemia both results from and encourages infection in the diabetic patient, and good control of the blood glucose concentration is an important aspect of their treatment.

FURTHER READING

Diabetes Control and Complications Trial Research Group. The effect of intensive treatment of diabetes on the development and progression of long-term complications in insulin-dependent diabetes mellitus. N Engl J Med 1993; **329:** 977-86.

Greene DA, Lattimer SA, Sima AA. Sorbitol, phosphoinositides, and sodium-potassium-ATPase in the pathogenesis of diabetic complications. N Engl J Med 1987; **316:** 599-606.

Heart Protection Study Collaborative Group. MRC/BHF Heart Protection Study of cholesterol lowering with simvastatin in 20536 high-risk individuals: a randomised placebo-controlled trial. Lancet 2002; **360:** 7-22.

Heart Protection Study Collaborative Group. MRC/BHF Heart Protection Study of cholesterol lowering with simvastatin in 5963 people with diabetes: a randomised placebo-controlled trial. Lancet 2003; **361:** 2005-16.

Mogensen CE, Keane WF, Bennett PH *et al*. Prevention of diabetic renal disease with special reference to microalbuminuria. Lancet 1995; **346:** 1080-4.

Koskinen P, Mänttäri M, Manninen V *et al*. Coronary heart disease incidence in NIDDM patients in the Helsinki Heart Study. Diabetes Care 1992; **15:** 820-5.

Pyörälä K, Pedersen TR, Kjekshus J *et al*. Cholesterol lowering with simvastatin improves prognosis of diabetic patients with coronary heart disease. A subgroup analysis of the Scandinavian Simvastatin Survival study. Diabetes Care 1997; **20:** 614-20.

Sacks FM, Pfeffer MA, Moye LA *et al*. The effect of pravastatin on coronary events after myocardial infarction in patients with average cholesterol levels (CARE). N Engl J Med 1996; **335:** 1001-31.

Stratton IM, Adler AI, Neil AW *et al*. Association of glycaemia with macrovascular and microvascular complications of type 2 diabetes (UKPDS 35). Brit Med J 2000; **321:** 405-12.

Taguchi T, Brownlee M. The biochemical mechanisms of diabetic tissue damage in Pickup JC & Williams G (eds). Textbook of Diabetes (3rd edn), 2003. Oxford: Blackwell Science, pp 47.1-47.17.

United Kingdom Prospective Diabetes Study. Intensive blood-glucose control with sulphonylureas or insulin compared with conventional treatment and risk of complications in patients with type 2 diabetes (UKPDS 33). Lancet 1998; **352:** 837-52.

## CLINICAL CASES

### HYPERLIPIDAEMIA

A 54 year old Asian man attended his family doctor's surgery complaining of an increase in the frequency of his angina during a spell of cold weather. He weighed 97 kg, his BMI was 30 kg/m$^2$ and BP 139/89. Medication: isosorbide mononitrate 20 mg t.d.s. and ramipril 10 mg once daily. He was asymptomatic. The family doctor requested a lipid profile. The results were:

| Analyte | Result |
|---|---|
| Serum total cholesterol (mmol/L) | 8.3 |
| triglyceride (mmol/L) | 17.0 |

The biochemistry laboratory suggested that the doctor should exclude diabetes as a cause of this dyslipidaemia. Further investigations included:

| Analyte | Result | Reference range |
|---|---|---|
| Random venous plasma glucose (mmol/L) | 15 | |
| HbA$_{1c}$ (%) | 8.6 | < 6.0 |

He was commenced on a calorie restricted diet. Three months later the investigations were repeated. The results were:

| Analyte | Result |
|---|---|
| Random venous plasma glucose (mmol/L) | 8.2 |
| HbA$_{1c}$ (%) | 6.4 |
| Serum total cholesterol (mmol/L) | 5.8 |
| triglyceride (mmol/L) | 4.3 |
| HDL cholesterol (mmol/L) | 0.89 |

The patient was continued on his diet and commenced on lipid lowering medication (a fibrate).

*POINTS:*

1. Raised total cholesterol and triglyceride concentrations are common at diagnosis of type 2 diabetes and a significant improvement of this dyslipidaemia frequently accompanies the commencement of a diabetic diet.

2. Other secondary causes of hyperlipidaemia include alcohol excess and hypothyroidism.

3. A total cholesterol concentration > 5.2 mmol/L in a patient with established cardiovascular disease, despite the introduction of a low fat diet for more than three months, warrants treatment with lipid-lowering medication. Diabetic patients often display raised triglyceride concentrations in addition to any raised cholesterol concentrations, so that a fibrate may be a suitable first line drug if cholesterol is only moderately elevated, particularly if HDL is low.

RENAL COMPLICATIONS

A 52 year old Afro-Caribbean man, whose type 2 diabetes had been diagnosed 11 years earlier, attended his family doctor for his diabetes review. His BMI was 28 kg/m$^2$ and BP 148/92. Medication: glibenclamide 15 mg o.d; metformin 500 mg t.d.s. On examination: background retinopathy and peripheral neuropathy (absent ankle jerks and loss of vibration sense).

| Analyte | Result | Reference range |
|---|---|---|
| Random venous plasma glucose (mmol/L) | 12.3 | |
| Serum fructosamine (µmol/L) | 320 | 200 - 280 |
| HbA$_{1c}$ (%) | 8.5 | < 6.0 |
| **Urinalysis:** | | |
| Glycosuria | | ++ |
| Proteinuria | | ++ |
| Ketonuria | | 0 |

He had been noted to have + proteinuria at his check-up six months earlier.

Further investigations were arranged :

| Analyte | Result | Reference range |
|---|---|---|
| Serum sodium (mmol/L) | 143 | 134 -146 |
| potassium (mmol/L) | 4.8 | 3.4 - 5.2 |
| urea (mmol/L) | 13.0 | 3.4 - 8.0 |
| creatinine (µmol/L) | 201 | 60 - 126 |
| 24 hr urinary protein excretion (g/L) | 0.06 | < 0.2 |
| Microbiology: | | |
| Mid-stream urine for culture: no growth detected | | |

In view of his renal impairment, metformin was contraindicated. His oral hypogly-caemics were discontinued and he was transferred onto insulin therapy. He was also commenced on an ACE inhibitor for hypertension.

Results at subsequent annual reviews were as follows

| Time from date proteinuria first noted (years) | 1 | 2 | 4 | 6 |
|---|---|---|---|---|
| Random venous plasma glucose (mmol/L) | 9.6 | 8.3 | 10.9 | 12.5 |
| Serum fructosamine (µmol/L) | 346 | | | |
| $HbA_{1c}$ (%) | 8.4 | 7.0 | 7.7 | 8.3 |
| Serum creatinine (µmol/L) | 243 | 251 | 402 | 563 |
| Proteinuria | ++ | ++ | +++ | +++ |
| BP | 140/98 | 142/88 | 140/92 | 152/95 |

POINTS:

1. Persistent proteinuria is suggestive of diabetic nephropathy. It is important to exclude other causes, the commonest of which is a urinary tract infection.

2. Diabetic nephropathy is unusual in the absence of other microvascular complications (e.g. retinopathy, neuropathy).

3. There is good evidence that ACE inhibitor therapy may slow the progression of nephropathy in type 1 diabetic patients. The evidence is less clear in patients with type 2 diabetes.

4. Proteinuria invalidates the use of fructosamine as an accurate marker of glycaemic control.

5. Diabetes is now the main reason for dialysis and transplantation in Europe. No ethnic group is spared and indeed, the prevalence of diabetic nephropathy shows a racial group difference, being 2.5 times more frequent in Afro-Caribbeans than in Caucasians.

6. The ACE inhibitor was clearly insufficient to control the hypertension and treatment with additional agents would have been warrented.

MICROALBUMINURIA

A 33 year old Caucasian woman was seen in the annual review clinic. Type 1 diabetes had been diagnosed 13 years earlier. She was asymptomatic. Medication: Mixtard insulin 30/70, 24 units mane, 14 units nocte. Her BP was 162/92. Fundoscopy revealed background retinopathy, which had been stable for two years. She had been noted to have proteinuria on one previous occasion nine months earlier.

Results:

| Analyte | Result | Reference range |
|---|---|---|
| Random venous plasma glucose (mmol/L) | 7.9 | |
| $HbA_{1c}$ (%) | 6.3 | < 6.0 |
| Glycosuria | 0 | |
| Proteinuria | + | |
| Urine protein (mg/L) | 165 | 20 - 200 |

Microbiology:
Mid-stream urine for culture: no growth detected

She was commenced on an ACE inhibitor.

Subsequent results were as follows:

| Date | July 1996 | February 1997 | August 1997 |
|---|---|---|---|
| Random venous plasma glucose (mmol/L) | 6.8 | 8.9 | 9.3 |
| HbA$_{1c}$ (%) | 6.2 | 9.6 | 6.0 |
| Urine protein (mg/L) | 162 | 195 | 170 |

*POINTS*

1. Patients with intermittent proteinuria should be investigated for microalbuminuria

2. There is good evidence that ACE inhibitor therapy may delay the progression of microalbuminuria in type 1 diabetic patients.

3. Microalbuminuria is a non-specific marker for diabetic nephropathy. Any systemic inflammatory condition will result in microalbuminuria owing to renal capillary leakage of plasma proteins. In February 1997 the patient was complaining of a respiratory tract infection, which may have increased her proteinuria temporarily.

# Chapter 7

# The role of clinical biochemistry in the diabetes clinic

The findings of both the Diabetes Control and Complications Trial (DCCT) for type 1 diabetes mellitus and the United Kingdom Prospective Diabetes Study (UKPDS) for type 2 diabetes can be summarised as having shown that good glycaemic control prevents or delays the development of microvascular and neuropathic complications. It may also have a beneficial effect upon macrovascular complications.

All patients with diagnosed diabetes are on treatment, whether by diet alone or diet combined with oral hypoglycaemic agents or insulin. As such, their treatment and progress must be monitored. The frequency with which they are seen by medical or specialist nursing staff and other health professionals will be dependent on the stability of their disease, the existence of complications and any special needs. At times of poor control, patients may need to be seen frequently. When apparently well controlled and free of complications, an annual review may be sufficient. However, the UKPDS recommendation is that to achieve an optimum degree of control, it is probably necessary to assess patients more frequently. In practice, this is often achieved through shared care arrangements with primary care physicians and practice nurses

## THE HOSPITAL DIABETES CLINIC

Traditionally, formal diabetes clinics have been held in hospitals, where the variety of specialist expertise required to support the diabetes physician and specialist nurse is readily available. Such expertise includes dietetics, ophthalmology, chiropody and laboratory services, particularly clinical biochemistry. Easy access to renal medicine and cardiology services are also important, the latter because of the importance of diabetes as a major risk factor for cardiovascular disease.

Most hospitals will have several diabetes clinic sessions each week. A structured approach to the organisation of diabetes care in the clinic setting makes it simpler for the professionals involved, and more appropriate for the needs of individual patients. One approach is to organise the clinics so that each deals with patients with particular problems. For example, there may be an annual review clinic for those with well-controlled diabetes, a 'new patient' clinic, a paediatric diabetes clinic, a clinic for those with diabetes in pregnancy and clinics run in conjunction with other clinical specialties, for patients with, for example, nephropathy, retinopathy or dyslipidaemia.

| The role of the hospital diabetes clinic |
| --- |
| 1. Diagnosis/confirmation of the diagnosis of diabetes |
| 2. Initiation of treatment |
| 3. Monitoring and changing treatment |
| 4. Annual review/screening for complications |
| 5. Monitoring complications. |

**Figure 7.1 The role of the hospital diabetes clinic**

## CLINICAL BIOCHEMISTRY AND THE CLINIC

All diabetes clinics require input from the clinical biochemistry department. Exactly how this support is given will be dependent on local circumstances, and the level of support, in terms of the repertoire of analyses offered, may differ depending on the type of clinic. Up-to-date biochemistry results should be available to diabetes physicians when they see patients, to facilitate early decisions on therapy and further referral when appropriate. The challenge for the laboratory is to make these results available when required, with minimal disruption to the lives of patients and the running of the diabetes clinic.

There are several ways by which this can be achieved:

• arranging for blood to be taken from the patient a few days before the clinic, perhaps in the family doctor's surgery, then forwarded to the laboratory for analysis

• sending capillary blood specimens or filter paper blood spots to the laboratory for glycated haemoglobin measurement prior to the clinic

• provision of an on-site service, either in the clinic or by fast tracking through the main laboratory.

The availability of laboratory results on ward and clinic computer terminals makes approaches which require specimens to be sent for analysis prior to the patient's appointment date and performing the analyses in a remote laboratory more feasible than they used to be.

In most diabetes clinics, at least some biochemistry analyses are available in 'real-time'. This may vary from blood glucose measurements by meter, probably performed by clinic nursing staff, to an extensive biochemistry service with a range of analyses, run by laboratory staff. When specimens are analysed in the clinic, it is vital that there is a fail-safe method for marrying up the results with the patients' notes.

DIAGNOSIS

Part of the work of a hospital diabetes service will be to confirm the diagnosis of the disease. The clinical biochemistry department is likely to be involved in the performance of glucose tolerance tests and this may well be in the clinic setting, according to local circumstances. The diagnosis of diabetes and the role of the laboratory in this is covered elsewhere in this book and will not be dealt with further here.

MONITORING OF GLYCAEMIC CONTROL

*BLOOD GLUCOSE*

For many years, glycaemic control was assessed in the diabetes clinic by measuring patients' blood glucose concentrations. This was because there was little else that could be measured that was recognised as being relevant to the disease. Now, its measurement in the clinic is of less importance given that many patients are able to self-monitor, usually quantitatively, and that provided the testing is carried out correctly (an important caveat), a clear picture of blood glucose control during the day can be obtained from these records.

However, on many occasions there is a marked discrepancy between the degree of control suggested by home blood glucose monitoring results and that indicated by glycated protein values obtained in the laboratory. Possible reasons include poor meter technique, inaccurate recording of results and, sometimes, deliberate fabrication of results. The availability of meters with built-in memory facilities that can store results may reveal the cause of such discrepancies.

Another factor that we have found in our clinic is that doctors seem more likely to make changes to therapy when a glycated protein concentration indicates poor control if there is an elevated random glucose value as well. The availability of blood glucose measurement in the clinic appears to provide some reassurance to the doctor that intervention is required.

If glucose measurement is not routinely performed on all patients attending the clinic, it should be available for certain circumstances, such as when there is concern about the development of ketoacidosis. If ketones are detected in the urine, blood glucose measurement is mandatory.

*GLYCATED PROTEINS*

Because of the findings in DCCT and UKPDS that there is a direct relationship between poor control and the development of complications, biochemical parameters that provide an index of diabetic control over a period of time are by far the most important analyses to have available in the clinic. All such assays are based on the measurement of a glycated protein, usually haemoglobin. However, glycated plasma proteins, measured as fructosamine, have also been used for this purpose.

The theory underlying their usefulness is that glucose attaches to the amino groups of proteins non-enzymatically and that the proportion of the protein becoming glycated is dependent on the prevailing glucose concentration over the lifespan of the protein. The poorer the overall diabetic control, the greater the amount of protein that becomes glycated.

*Haemoglobin $A_{1c}$*

The glycated protein that was used to assess control in the US and UK trials was haemoglobin $A_{1c}$, which is specifically haemoglobin $A_0$ that has been modified post-translationally by the process described above so that a glucose molecule is attached to the N-terminal valine residue of the $\alpha$-chain. Results are expressed as a percentage of total haemoglobin. The Diabetes National Framework Standards Document specifically identifies measurement of $HbA_{1c}$ as the analysis that should be available to all people with diabetes to monitor their glycaemic control.

The problem with $HbA_{1c}$ measurement has been in the standardisation of the results. Many different techniques are used for its measurement, including HPLC based systems, immunoassays and affinity chromatography, and reference ranges vary widely. Results obtained using one analytical system are not comparable with those obtained using others. This problem is well recognised in the specialties of clinical biochemistry and diabetes, and there are expert groups in Europe, the USA and Japan that are examining the issue, which is also being considered by an expert panel of the International Federation of Clinical Chemistry (IFCC).

Both the DCCT and UKPDS trials related their results to a specific HPLC method for $HbA_{1c}$ that was used initially for the DCCT trial, so direct comparisons can be made between the $HbA_{1c}$ figures recommended as indicative of good diabetic control for type 1 and type 2 diabetes. In the USA, considerable work has been done in adopting the use of the DCCT method as the primary standard for $HbA_{1c}$ measurement. This has been made possible by close liaison between the American Association of Clinical Chemistry (AACC) and the American Diabetes Association (ADA). Clinical laboratories in the USA can participate in a quality assurance scheme that enables them to check their calibration against the DCCT's recommendations.

Much of the responsibility for achieving standardisation across methodologies for $HbA_{1c}$ must now rest with the manufacturers of reagents and analytical systems. Many of these are 'closed' systems, where it is impossible for the user to modify parameters fixed on purchase. In the USA, where new reagent systems must be approved by the Federal Drug Administration (FDA) prior to being launched onto the market, only those systems that comply with the DCCT standardisation are now being licensed. There is considerable pressure for universal agreement on standardisation. The International Federation of Clinical Chemistry (IFCC) has established a reference method for $HbA_{1c}$, standardisation of which is based on pure $HbA_0$ and pure $HbA_{1c}$. From January 2004, this method has been used for the calibration of all methods used for $HbA_{1c}$ measurement in the European Union, to ensure conformity with the *In Vitro* Diagnostic Medical Device (IVD) Directive. Results obtained using IFCC calibration are significantly lower than DCCT values, and to prevent confusion clinically, $HbA_{1c}$ results will continue to be reported as DCCT-aligned values in the immediate future in the UK, although this practice will be kept under review.

Although most analytical systems available for glycated haemoglobin analysis measure true $HbA_{1c}$, there are techniques, once widely used, which measure total $HbA_1$, in which molecules other than glucose are attached to the N-terminal valine group of the $\alpha$-chain. An example is urea, which will attach to the same amino groups, forming carbamylated haemoglobin. High concentrations of urea are found in patients with renal failure, making total $HbA_1$ an unsuitable index of control in patients with diabetic renal disease. Techniques based on electroendosmosis on agarose gel separate $HbA_1$, not $HbA_{1c}$, from the other fractions, thus limiting their utility.

When interpreting glycated haemoglobin results, the scientist or clinician must always be aware of the potential for misleading results to be obtained in the presence of variant haemoglobins such as HbS, HbF, etc. These variant haemoglobins behave in different ways to HbA in the various analytical systems. For example, in immunologically based methods, the potential for interference will depend on the cross-reactivity characteristics of the antiserum. In general, HPLC methods are more discriminating in their ability to identify variant haemoglobins.

The lifespan of a red cell is approximately 120 days. Glycated haemoglobin measurements therefore assess diabetic control over a relatively clearly defined period of 6-8 weeks. However, where there is an abnormally fast turnover of red cells, such as in haemolytic anaemias, measurements reflect control over a shorter period.

*Other glycated proteins*

Attempts have been made to use other individual glycated proteins, which have shorter half lives, as indices of diabetic control over a shorter time period. Such an index would in theory be valuable in certain circumstances, such as in pregnancy, but so far their use has been limited. However, the measurement of fructosamine, which is essentially a measure of total glycated plasma protein, has been extensively studied. Fructosamine gives an indication of control over a 3-4 week period.

The major contributor to fructosamine values is glycated albumin. However, it has been established that other proteins, and possibly non-protein components, contribute to the values obtained. Standardisation of the assay has been difficult and most laboratories rely on the manufacturers of their chosen reagent system to establish correct calibration. Fructosamine has certain advantages in that it can be measured alongside other serum parameters on standard clinical laboratory analysers and does not necessitate an additional whole blood specimen, seperate instrumentation and additional laboratory technical time. However, it is now generally only measured in a few circumstances, for example, in haemolytic anaemias, which invalidate $HbA_{1c}$ measurements.

There are some clinical situations where fructosamine measurements will not provide useful information, for example, when there is a significant increase in protein turnover. In diabetes, this most frequently occurs as a result of proteinuria in patients with nephropathy. Also, it should be remembered that an inverse relationship exists between weight and fructosamine concentration. In obese patients, fructosamine concentrations are lower than expected for the degree of control. Figure 7.2 shows the relationship between fructosamine concentration and body weight in over 200 newly diagnosed people with type 2 diabetes. In summary, specific measurement of $HbA_{1c}$ remains the gold standard among glycated proteins for assessing glycaemic control.

Glycated protein measurements in patients with diabetes provide the best available information about recent glycaemic control, and together with knowledge of blood glucose concentrations throughout the day and their relationship to food intake and insulin or other therapy regime, may help the clinician make decisions on treatment adjustment to improve control. At present, however, their measurement has no role in the diagnosis of diabetes.

**Relationship of fructosamine and body weight**

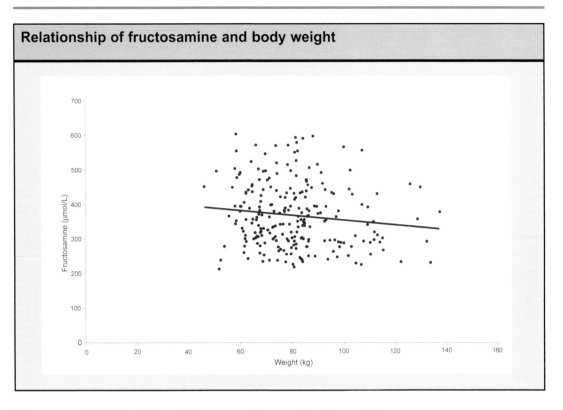

**Figure 7.2 Relationship of fructosamine and body weight**

## CLINICAL BIOCHEMISTRY AND THE ANNUAL REVIEW CLINIC

The function of the annual review clinic is to screen for the micro- and macrovascular complications of diabetes, which are associated with high morbidity and mortality. Clinical biochemistry has an important contribution to make to this process. First, some overall measure of glycaemic control is needed as described above. In addition, since it is recognised that diabetic patients benefit from treatment of abnormal lipids to a similar extent as non-diabetic patients, lipid measurements should also be performed at the annual review clinic. The early detection of abnormal albumin excretion is also important, through measurement of microalbuminuria (see below) for identifying patients at high risk of both renal and cardiovascular disease, and for prompting therapeutic intervention.

*MICROVASCULAR COMPLICATIONS*

The detection and monitoring of proteinuria forms an essential part of the review process for patients with diabetes. Subjecting urine to testing with 'Albustix' is of limited use in diabetic patients. The poor sensitivity of the method allows it to detect only relatively large amounts of protein, corresponding to a 24-hour excretion greater than 250 mg, defined as clinical proteinuria. The excretion of albumin in normal subjects is less than 20 mg/24h. The ability to measure concentrations of albumin in urine that indicate rates of excretion between these two extremes, so-called microalbuminuria, is extremely important.

Microalbuminuria appears to be a good prognostic indicator of the future development of diabetic complications. The detection of microalbuminuria in a diabetic patient may not solely indicate the development of renal impairment, although in type 1 diabetes it probably does if other causes are excluded. In type 2 diabetes, it is also a risk marker for cardiovascular disease. Excellent blood glucose control seems to abolish microalbuminuria in some instances and the findings of both the DCCT and UKPDS confirm that tight control can slow down or prevent the progression to clinical (Albustix +ve) proteinuria and chronic renal disease.

When microalbuminuria is first revealed by a screening test (usually measurement of urinary albumin:creatinine ratio, see below), the possibility of other causes of proteinuria must be considered. These include physiological causes, e.g. exercise; pathophysiological causes, e.g. hyperglycaemia, and pathological causes, e.g. urinary tract infection. If these factors are excluded, the patient should be retested to confirm the presence of microalbuminuria. If a second test is positive, a timed urine sample should be collected for measurement of the albumin excretion rate (AER). If this is less than 20 µg/min, no immediate action is required, but the patient should be retested, usually a year later. If the AER is greater than 20 µg/min, two further samples should be obtained. If the AER is greater than 20 µg/min in either of these, the patient must be carefully monitored, and steps taken to reduce the risk of progression to diabetic nephropathy. Adequate control of blood pressure is of major importance and current practice in type 1 diabetic patients is to use ACE inhibitors, which seem to have an additional reno-protective effect over and above their effects upon blood pressure. Their use may be appropriate even in the absence of hypertension if microalbuminuria is present.

For screening purposes, the albumin:creatinine ratio in a random urine sample has been shown to correlate well with AER values calculated from timed overnight urine collections. Using this ratio removes the necessity for accurate timing, but the introduction of a second assay (urine creatinine) provides increased opportunity for error. The methods for measuring albumin are immunologically based, using antiserum specific to human albumin. Semi-quantitative 'stick'-based methods, which can be used at the point of care, are now available and can be used in the clinic for screening in those patients recognised as being particularly at risk of developing complications. However, positive or borderline results should always be followed up by laboratory measurement of albumin in an accurately timed urine collection or of the AER. A timed overnight urine specimen for microalbumin measurement and calculation of AER is easier for the patient than making a 24 h collection and minimises the contribution of exercise-induced albumin excretion to the measurement.

In patients with established renal disease, other biochemical tests, such as plasma creatinine and potassium, will also be required to monitor the effects of renal insufficiency. It should be remembered that measurement of plasma creatinine concentration is of no value in detecting early renal dysfunction although, once elevated, it becomes a sensitive indicator of declining renal function.

*MACROVASCULAR COMPLICATIONS*
Most people with diabetes mellitus will die of the macrovascular complications of the disease. Along with hypertension, cigarette smoking and abnormal blood lipids, diabetes mellitus is a major risk factor for vascular (principally coronary, but also peripheral and cerebrovascular) disease. Antihypertensive and lipid-lowering therapies are frequently indicated in diabetic patients in an attempt to slow down the development of cardiovascular disease and peripheral vascular disease.

The measurement of total cholesterol, HDL-cholesterol and triglycerides in patients attending the diabetic clinic is essential to assess the need for treatment and to monitor it when it has been instituted. Dietary counselling for patients with diabetes includes advice on low fat diets.

## ANALYSERS FOR THE CLINIC
In recent years, several analytical systems suitable for clinic use have been introduced to the market. Systems for $HbA_{1C}$ and microalbumin measurements are ideally suited for use in the clinic, as minimal specimen preparation is required and clinically important results for patients with diabetes are available rapidly. Some of these systems are simple to use and can be operated by appropriately trained non-laboratory personnel but, as for blood glucose meters, there must be appropriate input from the laboratory with respect to training and quality assurance.

## OTHER BIOCHEMISTRY REQUIREMENTS
The range of biochemical tests required on a regular basis, with a relatively rapid turnaround, for patients attending the diabetes clinic is relatively small, comprising measures of glycaemic control, renal impairment and lipid status. However, in certain circumstances, other analyses will be required, although not necessarily on a real-time basis. For example, where new therapies are introduced, with the possibility of side-effects, routine measurement of renal function or liver function tests may be indicated.

## DIABETES RESOURCE CENTRES

Hospital diabetes clinics are often held in, or associated with Diabetes Resource Centres, which are run as multidisciplinary units. The first-line contact for the patient or the referring doctor is usually the diabetes specialist nurse, whose prime role is educating patients with diabetes about their disease and instructing them in all aspects of living with diabetes, such as blood glucose monitoring, administration of insulin and other hypoglycaemic agents, weight control, and general counselling and advice. The Resource Centre nurses have direct access to medical staff specialising in diabetes, dieticians and chiropodists. They also have close links with clinical biochemistry staff, particularly in the area of blood glucose monitoring.

There is a real clinical governance issue surrounding the correct use of blood glucose meters. It is vitally important that there are intensive, ongoing training arrangements for users, whether health professionals or people with diabetes. If used correctly, they provide valuable information about control on which changes to treatment can be based. Used incorrectly, results generated can lead to inappropriate treatment, usually with glucose or insulin, which has led to fatalities.

Training is usually organised on a collaborative basis with the meter manufacturer. In a hospital setting, this will involve liaison between the laboratory and specialist diabetes nurses to identify areas where meters are to be located and to organise training sessions for staff who will be using them. Because of working arrangements, it is usually necessary to arrange training sessions both in the daytime and in the evening. Best practice dictates that only when the trainer is satisfied that an individual is competent in the use and care of the meter can he or she become a designated user. Training should include basic instruction in quality control techniques as well as the importance of correct storage of reagent strips and quality control materials, and not exceeding expiry dates. The most common problem encountered is that insufficient blood is added to the reagent pad, and training in meter use must include instructions on capillary blood sampling.

A register should be kept of designated users. Some suppliers of meters provide certificates of competence that can be issued to staff on the successful completion of training.

It is sensible to have a named contact in clinical areas that have blood glucose meters. This person should be responsible for keeping the register of designated users up to date, ensuring that quality assurance procedures are followed, arranging for new staff to be trained and reporting problems. The first-line contact is likely to be a member of the laboratory staff.

The UK Joint Working Group on Quality Assurance has issued revised guidelines on point of care testing, reiterating the importance of clinical laboratory involvement in ensuring the quality of such services. Where there is a hospital-wide policy on blood glucose monitoring, it is usual for the diabetes specialist nurses and laboratory staff to work together in the selection of meters, training of ward staff and implementation and monitoring of both internal quality control and external quality assessment. Training and quality aspects are often dealt with in close collaboration with the meter manufacturer.

Clinical Pathology Accreditation (UK) Ltd recognises the importance of clinical laboratory involvement in the support of extra-laboratory instrumentation and excludes areas where testing is done without this support from the accreditation status of the main laboratory. The impact of clinical governance initiatives in the NHS is likely to increase the involvement of hospital laboratories in the provision of appropriate point of care testing arrangements in all clinical areas.

## DIABETES CLINICS IN PRIMARY CARE
Increasing numbers of primary care practices now undertake diabetes clinics for their patients, particularly for those with type 2 diabetes mellitus. Practice nurses are usually closely involved in the running of these clinics and links to the diabetes nurse specialists at the Diabetes Resource Centre are to be encouraged.

The range of biochemistry analyses required for primary care clinics is, of course, the same as that required for patients attending a hospital diabetes clinic. At the present time, it is unlikely that a near-patient testing facility capable of providing all these analyses on a real-time basis, in an economically viable way, is feasible. However, some analyses, for example, $HbA_{1c}$ and microalbumin measured using the dedicated systems mentioned earlier, could be used by appropriately trained personnel in primary care. It may well be that, in the future, clinical laboratory staff will become more involved in supporting such ventures, analogous to the support already provided for blood glucose monitoring in the community by some laboratories.

## SHARED DIABETES CARE
The concept of shared care between the general practitioner and the hospital diabetes specialist provides the opportunity, particularly for well controlled patients, to have routine monitoring performed locally, at their primary care surgery; it also provides the family doctor with access to advice from the diabetes specialist should problems arise, and educational support for practice staff having responsibility for the care of patients with diabetes. In most cases, patients who are to be treated with insulin will attend the hospital diabetes centre for education and for their insulin regimen to be stabilised.

It is inevitable that the involvement of primary care practitioners in the monitoring and care of people with diabetes will increase. A more sedentary lifestyle and an increasingly obese population has led to a significant increase in the number of people diagnosed with type 2 diabetes in Western societies. It is recognised in the UK that many remain undiagnosed and a major campaign to raise public awareness of diabetes is underway.

The additional healthcare resources required to support these increased numbers of patients and optimise their diabetic control in order to minimise the risk of long term complications will be directed to primary care. Alongside this, the various National Service Frameworks for Diabetes for the countries of the UK have made recommendations for biochemical monitoring and its frequency. Together with initiatives such as the General Medical Services contract in England and Wales, which gives family doctors targets based on the achievement of satisfactory $HbA_{1c}$ levels in patients with diabetes, this will inevitably lead to increased biochemistry testing. Initially, the additional work will be absorbed by hospital clinical biochemistry laboratories but, in time, increased provision of point of care testing is likely to have an important role.

## FURTHER READING

John WG. Glycated haemoglobin analysis. Ann Clin Biochem 1997; **34:** 153-63.

Marshall SM, Barth JH. Standardisation of HbA1c measurement: a concensus statement. Ann Clin Biochem 2000; **37:** 45-6.

Marshall SM, Home PD, Manley SE, Barth JH, John WG. Standardisation of glycated haemoglobin. Ann Clin Biochem 2002; **39:** 78-9.

Willekens E, Thienpont L, Stöckl D, Kobold U, Weiland H, De Leenheer AP. Quantification of glycohemoglobin on blood by mass spectrometry applying multiple-reaction monitoring. Clin Chem 2000; **46:** 281-83.

Bry L, Chen P, Sacks DB. Effects of hemoglobin variants and chemically modified derivatives on assays for glycohemoglobin. Clin Chem 2001; **47:** 153-63.

## CLINICAL CASES

### OBESE PERSON WITH RAISED HbA$_{1c}$ AND LOW FRUCTOSAMINE

In May 1997, a 58 year old man with type 2 diabetes mellitus attended his six-monthly diabetes review at his family doctor's surgery. He mentioned that he had felt lethargic for the past few months and complained of nocturia, but had not had other symptoms. Diabetes had been diagnosed four years earlier. He weighed 104 kg; his BMI was 34 kg/m$^2$. His medication consisted of glibenclamide 15 mg o.d. and metformin 850 mg t.d.s. He performed no home glucose monitoring and had no evidence of diabetic complications.

His biochemistry results had been as follows:

| Date | Random plasma glucose mmol/L | Fructosamine μmol/L |
|---|---|---|
| May 1997 | 13.6 | 330 |
| November 1997 | 11.0 | 318 |
| May 1998 | 12.6 | 312 |
| No proteinuria was detected on urinalysis. | | |

Although the patient's fructosamine concentration was outside the non-diabetic range (200-280 μmol/L) that corresponds to good control, it had previously been only slightly elevated. At the same time, the patient was reluctant to convert to insulin therapy, as would be indicated should control not prove to be adequate. To confirm that diabetic control was poor, the family doctor requested HbA$_{1c}$ be measured: the result was 10.4% The patient was persuaded to change to insulin therapy.

Results after four months of treatment with insulin:

| Analyte | Result |
|---|---|
| Random plasma glucose (mmol/L) | 8.3 |
| Fructosamine (μmol/L) | 271 |
| HbA$_{1c}$ (%) | 7.0 |

*POINTS*

1. Fructosamine can be artefactually low in obese patients. In these patients, isolated measurements provide a poor indicator of absolute glycaemic control, but serial measurements can still be used to monitor glycaemic control in an individual patient whose BMI remained unchanged. $HbA_{1c}$ is a much better index of glycaemic control.

2. Insulin has an anabolic effect and usually results in some initial weight gain.

3. Conditions that lower plasma protein concentrations will also affect fructosamine concentrations and underestimate the level of glycaemia, e.g. proteinuria, catabolic states.

NORMAL GLUCOSE AND $HbA_{1c}$ BUT RAISED FRUCTOSAMINE CONCENTRATION

A 63 year old women with insulin treated type 2 diabetes attended for her diabetes annual review. She performed regular home blood glucose monitoring and this indicated good overall control of her diabetes, with no values > 10 mmol/L. She weighed 76 kg. She had noticed that she had lost some weight over the previous few months but did not complain of any osmotic symptoms.

| Analyte | Result | Reference range |
|---|---|---|
| Blood glucose (mmol/L) | 5.6 | |
| Serum fructosamine (µmol/L) | 401 | 200-280 |

The raised fructosamine concentration appeared surprising. It was therefore repeated and in addition a sample was taken for $HbA_{1c}$.

| Analyte | Result | Reference range |
|---|---|---|
| Fructosamine (µmol/L) | 405 | 200-280 |
| $HbA_{1c}$ (%) | 6.1 | 3.5-6.5 |

Further biochemistry tests were performed:

| Analyte | Result | Reference range |
|---|---|---|
| Serum albumin (g/L) | 32 | 34-51 |
| total protein (g/L) | 98 | 60-80 |

Serum protein electrophoresis displayed a monoclonal band with immunosuppression. Immunofixation confirmed a diagnosis of IgA myeloma

| Analyte | Result | Reference range |
|---|---|---|
| Serum IgA (g/L) | 8.2 | 0.65-3.75 |
| IgG (g/L) | 4.0 | 8.0-14.5 |
| IgM (g/L) | 0.5 | 0.2-3.0 |

*POINTS*

1. Patients' home blood glucose monitoring often suggests better control than is indicated by objective laboratory indices such as fructosamine and $HbA_{1c}$. Nevertheless, it is important to repeat and confirm any anomalous result.

2. Any clinical condition that significantly affects blood total protein concentration (e.g. myeloma, protein-losing nephropathies) will influence fructosamine concentration independently of glycaemic control.

MISLEADING GLYCATED PROTEIN RESULTS

A white male was diagnosed with diabetes in 1995 at the age of 58. Random plasma glucose was 19.3 mmol/L and serum fructosamine 458 μmol/L. He was treated with dietary energy restriction; three months later his fructosamine was 295 μmol/L. In October 1996, the local laboratory wrote to the family doctor stating that fructosamine measurement had been superseded by $HbA_{1c}$ measurement. They also reported results for the following (but did not comment on them):

| Analyte | Result | Reference range |
|---|---|---|
| Random glucose (mmol/L) | 12.3 | |
| Serum fructosamine (μmol/L) | 400 | 200-280 |
| $HBA_{1c}$ (%) | 3.1 | < 6.0 |

The family doctor recalled the patient and noted that he was jaundiced and that the liver was palpable below the costal margin. Further investigation revealed:

| Analyte | Result | Reference range |
|---|---|---|
| Hb (g/dL) | 10.0 | 11.5-18.0 |
| Platelets (x $10^9$/L) | 109 | 150-450 |
| Reticulocytes (%) | 35 | < 1 |
| Coombs' test negative | | |
| Serum bilirubin (μmol/L) | 73 | < 20 |
| ALT (IU/L) | 34 | < 35 |
| Alkaline phosphatase (IU/L) | 210 | 110-390 |

The blood film was reported as showing spherocytes ++ and further discussion with the patient at this stage elicited a history of congenital spherocytosis. His diabetic control (as assessed by fructosamine) was moderate and in 2000 he developed atrial flutter/fibrillation for which he was warfarinised. His urine, which had previously been negative for protein, tested positive for protein in 2000 and has been consistently positive since that time. His 24-hour urine collection showed a urinary albumin excretion of 1.14 g/L and a 24-hour excretion of 2.24 g/24h. Serum albumin concentration was 34 g/L. His most recent results show a plasma glucose of 18.7 mmol/L with a fructosamine of 280 μmol/L and a $HbA_{1c}$ of 5.1%.

*POINTS:*

1.  There are a number of explanations for apparent discrepancies between glucose results and glycated protein results and an explanation should always be sought. Haemolytic anaemia is one explanation of an artefactually low $HbA_{1c}$ although it is uncommon in everyday practice.

2.  Fructosamine results are profoundly influenced by proteinuria and low circulating albumin concentrations.

3.  It is unusual for both $HbA_{1c}$ and fructosamine measurements to be ineffective in the assessment of diabetic control.

# Chapter 8

# The management of diabetes in pregnancy

## INTRODUCTION

Diabetes mellitus is one of the most prevalent diseases that affects pregnant women. Established maternal type 1 or type 2 diabetes is present in 0.2-0.5% of all pregnancies and, in addition, gestational diabetes mellitus (GDM) complicates 1-3% of pregnancies.

Pregnancy in a woman with established diabetes is a high-risk condition, for both mother and baby, in the current pregnancy and in the future. It is associated with a higher rate of miscarriage, congenital malformations and stillbirth than pregnancy in non-diabetic women. The incidence of pregnancy-associated hypertension (pre-eclampsia), polyhydramnios, premature labour, maternal infection and ketoacidosis are all increased. In women in whom glycaemic control is poor, neonatal complications of hypoglycaemia, respiratory distress syndrome and jaundice occur more frequently, increasing perinatal morbidity and mortality. In the mother, significant deterioration of diabetic retinal and renal disease may occur, especially in women with long-standing disease. In pregnancy, the changing hormonal environment reduces glucose tolerance in normal women, though not usually to a significant extent. In women with diabetes, however, the effects of pregnancy are much greater and glycaemic control can differ considerably.

Gestational diabetes mellitus is defined as carbohydrate intolerance first identified during pregnancy, and although not associated with congenital abnormalities, is associated with increased risks of macrosomia, stillbirth and operative delivery.

An optimal outcome for the pregnancy requires the close collaboration of a team of medical and allied professionals, and extensive evidence is now available showing that a successful outcome is much more likely if normoglycaemia is achieved before and maintained during pregnancy.

## CLASSIFICATION

Some means of classifying maternal diabetes is valuable since it allows relation of outcome to a particular type of diabetes or abnormal glucose tolerance. A useful way of classifying diabetes in pregnancy is to consider it as present before pregnancy (pre-gestational) or developing in pregnancy (gestational diabetes) (*see Figure 8.1*). The new WHO diagnostic criteria have redefined gestational diabetes as any degree of glucose intolerance in pregnancy, thus including the previously separate category of gestational impaired glucose intolerance.

---

**Classification of maternal diabetes in pregnancy**

Pre-gestational diabetes mellitus

    a) type 1 diabetes diagnosed before pregnancy
    b) type 2 diabetes diagnosed before pregnancy
    c) impaired glucose tolerance (IGT) diagnosed before pregnancy

Gestational diabetes

    Any degree of glucose intolerance with onset or first recognition during pregnancy

---

**Figure 8.1 Classification of maternal diabetes in pregnancy**

## DIAGNOSIS AND SCREENING

Diabetes can sometimes present in pregnancy with the finding of a significantly elevated random plasma glucose concentration but in the majority of cases, the diagnosis is made on the basis of the response to a glucose challenge. Because fasting and post-prandial glucose concentrations are normally lower in the first trimester and the early part of the second trimester of pregnancy than in normal, non-pregnant women, their measurement is unreliable for diagnostic purposes. The WHO recommends that gestational diabetes should be diagnosed using a standard 75 g oral glucose tolerance test (OGTT), performed following an overnight fast. The recent changes to the diagnostic criteria apply to gestational diabetes as well, decreasing the diagnostic fasting venous plasma glucose concentration from 7.8 to 7.0 mmol/L. All women diagnosed as having gestational diabetes should have the OGTT repeated at least six weeks after delivery so that they can be correctly classified as having diabetes mellitus, impaired glucose tolerance, impaired fasting glycaemia or normal glucose tolerance in the non-pregnant state. Gestational diabetes is associated with increased risk of developing diabetes mellitus at a later date.

The situation regarding the diagnosis of gestational diabetes in the USA is less clear. While expert groups on GDM have proposed diagnosis based on the 75 g OGTT, the practice most widely used until recently involved screening using a 50 g glucose load and plasma glucose measurement at one hour. If that value exceeded 7.8 mmol/L, a three hour, 100 g OGTT was performed. However, the American Diabetes Association (ADA), in their annual position statement on diagnosis and classification in 2004, recommended that screening need no longer be performed in low risk women. Pregnant women are deemed 'low risk' of developing GDM if they fulfil all the following criteria:

• < 25 years of age

• normal body weight

• no family history of DM

• no history of abnormal glucose metabolism

• no history of poor obstetric outcome

• not members of an ethnic/racial group with a high prevalence of diabetes (e.g. Hispanic, African, native American).

Because even in normal women, glucose tolerance deteriorates progressively during pregnancy, gestational diabetes may develop at any time. For this reason, routine testing of urine for glucose is recommended throughout pregnancy and remains the basis of any screening programme. Whenever significant glycosuria (which depends on the type of test strips used) is detected, it is recommended that a blood sample be taken for random glucose measurement. These random measurements should also be made at the booking visit and at 28 weeks gestation. A 75 g OGTT should be performed if a fasting plasma glucose concentration exceeds 6.0 mmol/L or the post-prandial concentration exceeds 7.0 mmol/L.

The WHO guidelines on the diagnosis of diabetes mellitus state that it may be appropriate to screen women from high risk groups for GDM. These include those with a family history of diabetes, a history of glucose intolerance or previous large babies, those from high-risk ethnic groups and those with elevated fasting or random glucose concentrations. There is a case for screening such individuals during the first trimester, to detect previously undiagnosed diabetes mellitus, rather than waiting for 24-28 weeks, when gestational diabetes is usually screened for.

In the UK, the National Institute for Clinical Excellence (NICE) states that current evidence does not support *routine* screening for gestational diabetes.

## MONITORING OF THE DIABETIC MOTHER
Monitoring and the goals of treatment are the same whether the woman has established or gestational diabetes. The aim of intervention is to achieve a normal delivery of a healthy baby as close as possible to term. From the beginning, care is multidisciplinary and shared between primary and secondary care providers, all of whom

make important contributions. It is universally accepted that good control of blood glucose during pregnancy, combined with intensive antenatal care, reduces perinatal mortality.

## PRE-PREGNANCY MONITORING

The prevention of congenital malformations, a potential leading cause of perinatal morbidity and mortality in pregnancy in women with diabetes, requires effective pre-pregnancy care. Consequently, for those with established diabetes, intervention should begin prior to pregnancy. These women should be encouraged to seek pre-pregnancy counselling and plan pregnancy carefully. Most centres caring for pregnant women with diabetes have established pre-pregnancy clinics, and prospective studies have demonstrated that pre-conception counselling and improved glycaemic control reduces the incidence of congenital malformations.

Pre-pregnancy clinics give an opportunity to record detailed medical and obstetric histories and assess diabetic complications, particularly retinopathy and nephropathy. The goals of glycaemic control can be discussed and measures taken to work towards them. Reinforcement of dietary advice, if followed, helps the patient achieve optimal glycaemic control. The diet should allow 30-35 kcal/kg/day pre-pregnant body weight and contain high levels of complex carbohydrate (50% of total energy), high levels of soluble fibre (30-50 g/day) and low levels of saturated fats. If not already being done, home blood glucose monitoring should be initiated and folate treatment (0.4 mg/day for up to 12 weeks) commenced. Contraception can be discussed to ensure that pregnancy does not occur until glycaemic control is normalised (as determined by home glucose monitoring and regular measurement of glycated haemoglobin). Oral hypoglycaemic agents are not recommended during pregnancy and if normoglycaemia cannot be achieved by diet only in those with type 2 diabetes, treatment with insulin should be initiated before conception. Tight glycaemic control can be associated with an increased risk of hypoglycaemia. For this reason, the woman and her partner should be instructed on the use and administration of glucagon.

## MONITORING DURING PREGNANCY

Once pregnancy is confirmed, the woman can be transferred to the antenatal clinic for continued care. Women with diabetes not attending a pre-pregnancy clinic should be encouraged to book early for antenatal care. Throughout pregnancy, the woman is reviewed every two weeks until 36 weeks and weekly thereafter. At each visit, a diabetes specialist nurse and midwife should be available to provide support. Using her own blood glucose meter, each expectant mother is encouraged to record 4-6 blood glucose measurements every day, aiming for fasting blood glucose concentrations of 5.0-6.0 mmol/L and postprandial concentrations of 7.0 mmol/L. Most centres complement home blood glucose monitoring with monthly measurement of glycated haemoglobin.

Women with type 1 diabetes who have established retinopathy at their booking visit are at risk of undergoing significant deterioration of this complication during pregnancy. Reasons for this may include the rapid improvement in glycaemic control early in pregnancy in addition to changes in retinal blood flow and concentrations of hormones. For this reason, careful retinal examination using a mydriatic agent and, preferably, retinal photography should be done at booking and at least once in each trimester to monitor any changes in the severity of retinopathy and identify any need for laser treatment.

Other women with diabetes who need careful management are those with established nephropathy. Renal function needs careful assessment at the booking visit and at regular intervals thereafter using serum urea, creatinine and electrolytes in addition to 24 h urinary protein excretion and, if necessary, creatinine clearance. Careful monitoring for, and treatment of, hypertension is essential to prevent progression of the nephropathy and ensure a successful outcome for mother and baby.

## MONITORING OF THE MOTHER WITH GESTATIONAL DIABETES
The management of women with gestational diabetes is similar to that for women with established diabetes prior to pregnancy. Once GDM is confirmed, the woman is reviewed by the diabetes nurse specialist for education and implementation of home blood glucose monitoring, and by the dietitian for dietary intervention. She should be reviewed one week after modifying her diet and the results of home blood glucose monitoring should be evaluated. If, during this period, two or more blood glucose measurements exceed the stated goals (fasting blood glucose 5.0-6.0 mmol/L, post prandial blood glucose 7.0 mmol/L), then insulin should be commenced. This may take the form of a single dose of a long acting insulin with short-acting insulin before meals or a twice daily mixture of short and long acting insulins. Thereafter, management follows that of other women with diabetes.

## FETAL WELL-BEING AND SURVEILLANCE
Serial measurements of fetal growth and liquor volume are used to assess fetal well-being. This information is used to determine the optimum time for delivery, thus minimising the risks of prematurity. Fetal growth is determined by maternal-fetal nutrient transfer, which is dependent on fetal size, uterine blood flow and nutrient supply, all factors that can be influenced by maternal diabetes.

Ultrasound examination forms the basis of modern surveillance of the fetus. A booking scan confirms dates accurately and a detailed scan is performed at 20 weeks to screen for congenital malformations. Fetal growth is assessed using measurements of the head and abdomen every four weeks throughout the second trimester and fortnightly during the third trimester. Excessive fetal growth presents as an increase in abdominal circumference in relation to head circumference. It is due to increased hepatic glycogen storage and subcutaneous fat deposition secondary to poor maternal control of glycaemia, with subsequent fetal hyperinsulinaemia. Asymmetrical growth retardation, indicated by an inadequately increasing fetal abdominal circumference, is a feature of pregnancies complicated by diabetic vascular disease, particularly those complicated by nephropathy, retinopathy or pre-eclampsia. Uteroplacental insufficiency preferentially spares brain growth at the expense of reduced liver glycogen stores and subcutaneous fat deposition. Asymmetrical growth is associated with increased risk of intrauterine death, intra-partum hypoxia and neonatal complications.

The concept of the biophysical profile was developed by Manning in the 1980s. This is an ultrasound-based assessment of fetal well-being derived from fetal movement, fetal tone, fetal breathing movements, liquor volume and a non-stress test of cardiac variability, assessed by monitoring Doppler heart rate. Each parameter has a possible score of 1, 1.5 or 2, the higher score representing normality in each case. The lower the score, the higher the perinatal mortality. Doppler measurements of umbilical artery blood flow are helpful in cases of intrauterine growth retardation. Abnormal umbilical artery resistance appears to be a significant predictor of fetal compromise in diabetic pregnancy. Fetal well-being is also reflected by liquor volume. In diabetic pregnancy, the main concern is the development of polyhydramnios (four-quadrant liquor volume above the 90th centile for gestational age) and is usually associated with poor maternal glycaemic control, leading to fetal hyperglycaemia and polyuria. Congenital anomalies of the gastrointestinal tract must always be excluded as a cause by ultrasonography. Polyhydramnios can be associated with pre-term labour or premature rupture of membranes, unstable lie and cord prolapse. It is also associ-ated with an increased risk of stillbirth. Oligohydramnios is less common and usually represents either ruptured membranes or poor fetoplacental perfusion.

## MANAGEMENT OF LABOUR AND DELIVERY

The challenge to the team caring for the woman with diabetes is to conduct her labour and delivery in a manner similar to that of a non-diabetic mother, avoiding unnecessary intervention and ensuring the delivery of a healthy infant, without causing unnecessary risks to either the mother or child. Uncomplicated diabetic pregnancies can be allowed to continue to full term provided that:

- there has been good glycaemic control

- there is no clinical and/or ultrasonic evidence of macrosomia

- there is no clinical and/or ultrasonic evidence of polyhydramnios

- there is no evidence of fetoplacental dysfunction

- there are no other obstetric complications such as hypertension, pre-eclampsia, major placenta praevia or intrauterine growth retardation, which would indicate the need for delivery.

The fact that a woman has diabetes, either established prior to the pregnancy or gestational, should not influence the decision on how she should be delivered. The same obstetric factors that obtain in any pregnancy should determine this decision. Therefore, a spontaneous unassisted vaginal delivery should be encouraged whenever possible. Induction of labour may be necessary with the use of prostaglandin to effect effacement of an unfavourable cervix. After inserting the prostaglandin gel, it is important to monitor the fetal heart and uterine contractions, as prostaglandin-induced uterine hypertonia can cause significant fetal distress, resulting in fetal death. Difficult vaginal delivery and shoulder dystocia should always be anticipated.

If the woman does require delivery by Caesarean section, prophylactic antibiotics should be given. The risk of neonatal respiratory distress syndrome can be reduced by preventing neonatal hypoxia; an epidural anaesthetic is therefore preferred. If a general anaesthetic is required, a short induction-delivery interval should minimise adverse changes to the Apgar score. A paediatrician should be at the delivery for all women with diabetes because of the physical and biochemical problems that may be encountered by the neonate.

Following spontaneous onset or induction, the management of labour, with the exception of the medical management of the woman's diabetes, is similar to that of any high risk pregnancy. The principal objective is to maintain maternal euglycaemia, as maternal hyperglycaemia can cause neonatal hypoglycaemia. An insulin and glucose infusion is used during labour to meet energy needs and to prevent the development of diabetic ketoacidosis. A constant 10% dextrose infusion of 100 mL per hour (10 g/hour) is used with a variable infusion rate of soluble insulin. Blood glucose concentration is monitored hourly and the insulin infusion adjusted to maintain a blood glucose concentration of 4.0-6.0 mmol/L (*Figure 8.2*).

| Guidelines for insulin infusion during labour and delivery | |
| --- | --- |
| Capillary blood glucose (mmol/L) | Insulin infusion rate (units/h) |
| <4.0 | 0 |
| 4-5.5 | 0.5 |
| 5.6-7.7 | 1.0 |
| 7.8-10 | 1.5 |
| 10.1-12.2 | 2.0 |
| >12.2 | 2.5 |

**Figure 8.2 Guidelines for insulin infusion during labour and delivery**

If the woman is to undergo a planned induction, the morning insulin should be withheld and an intravenous infusion of 5% dextrose commenced as early as possible, particularly if she has been given long acting insulin the night before. For those being delivered by elective Caesarean section, the operation should ideally be scheduled early in the morning, to minimise unnecessary maternal metabolic disturbances, which may have consequences for the fetus.

Fetal distress is more common in diabetic than non-diabetic pregnancies and for this reason fetal heart rate monitoring and fetal blood sampling should be routinely available during labour for all diabetic women. Following delivery, the insulin infusion rate should be halved immediately, as a rapid decline in insulin resistance follows delivery of the placenta. Once a normal diet has been resumed, the woman should revert to her pre-pregnancy insulin requirements. Breast feeding reduces insulin requirements by approximately 25% and an appropriate reduction in the dose should be made once lactation has become established.

## BIOCHEMICAL PROBLEMS OF THE NEONATE (*Figure 8.3*)
Following delivery, the baby should ideally remain with its mother to facilitate bonding and encourage breast feeding. Only if a neonatal problem is apparent or anticipated is neonatal unit care required. The main problems that may occur in the neonate are hypoglycaemia, respiratory distress syndrome, hypocalcaemia, polycythaemia and hyperbilirubinaemia.

| Perinatal problems affecting the infant of the diabetic mother |
|---|
| • Birth injury |
| • Asphyxia neonatorum |
| • Congenital malformation |
| • Hypoglycaemia |
| • Hypocalcaemia |
| • Hyperbilirubinaemia |
| • Polycythaemia |

Figure 8.3 Perinatal problems affecting the infant of the diabetic mother

NEONATAL HYPOGLYCAEMIA

Neonatal hypoglycaemia in the infants of diabetic mothers has been recognised for many years and the Pederson hypothesis explains the phenomenon. Maternal hyperglycaemia results in the sequence of fetal hyperglycaemia and consequent fetal hyperinsulinaemia that causes suppression of glycogenolysis and gluconeogenesis, resulting in neonatal hypoglycaemia. An early postnatal fall in blood glucose concentrations is an almost universal finding in neonates and is unlikely to be of pathological significance. Low blood glucose concentrations can even persist beyond this period in breast-fed infants of non-diabetic mothers but such infants mount an effective counter-regulatory hormonal response, which prompts ketone body formation, thus providing alternative fuels for cerebral metabolism. Therefore, the diagnosis of pathological hypoglycaemia in the infant of a diabetic mother requires the demonstration of its persistence beyond the first few postnatal hours, associated with a failure to mount a lipolytic and ketogenic response. The main clinical concern relating to neonatal hypoglycaemia is the risk of neurological damage, although there are no prospective controlled studies that have addressed this issue.

In view of the potential adverse neurological effects of neonatal hypoglycaemia, routine neonatal blood glucose monitoring should be performed for the first 24 hours after delivery. The first assessment is made following delivery, then hourly for three hours and subsequently every six hours until 24 hours. Not all infants of diabetic mothers will become hypoglycaemic and if early blood glucose concentrations are satisfactory, monitoring should be discontinued. Blood glucose test strips are inaccurate at low concentrations and if a measurement of < 4.0 mmol/L is obtained, a confirmatory blood or plasma glucose should be measured in the laboratory. The initial management of an otherwise healthy infant should consist of early and regular enteral feeds. If blood glucose concentrations remain low in two consecutive pre-feed measurements, despite optimising enteral intakes, or if the baby is symptomatic (fits or reduced level of consciousness), intravenous dextrose should be commenced at an infusion rate of 6-10 mg/kg/min, which can be reduced once euglycaemia is restored. A sustained blood glucose of < 2.2 mmol/L on the first day or < 2.6 mmol/L subsequently should be treated with an intravenous dextrose infusion even in the absence of symptoms. Enteral feeds should not be discontinued or reduced when intravenous glucose is commenced, unless the baby has other complications that put it at risk of fluid overload, such as congenital heart disease. As the baby recovers its glucose control, the rate of intravenous glucose infusion can be gradually reduced.

RESPIRATORY COMPLICATIONS
Infants of mothers with diabetes mellitus are at greater risk of respiratory distress syndrome (RDS) and transient tachypnoea of the newborn than infants of mothers without diabetes. The incidence of respiratory distress syndrome is reduced with good control of the maternal diabetes but other factors, such as Caesarean section, contribute. The incidence of RDS is about twice as great following delivery by section than after vaginal delivery.

Insulin inhibits cortisol-induced lecithin synthesis, probably by inhibiting the production of fibroblast-pneumocyte factor, which promotes phosphatidylcholine synthesis. In addition, high glucose concentrations inhibit the incorporation of choline into phosphatidylcholine, and butyrate inhibits the transcription of mRNA for surfactant proteins. These mechanisms contribute to surfactant deficiency and the increased incidence of RDS in infants of diabetic mothers. To minimise respiratory complications, one should aim to deliver the infant as close to term as possible. If pre-term delivery is indicated, corticosteroids should be administered early to enhance fetal lung maturity, with appropriate safeguards to prevent severe maternal hyperglycaemia and possible ketoacidosis. Surfactant should be administered early if the baby develops symptoms of respiratory distress syndrome.

HYPOCALCAEMIA
Hypocalcaemia in the newborn results from maternal urinary magnesium loss. This magnesium deficiency inhibits the recovery of parathyroid hormone concentrations (which fall and then rise in the normal neonate after birth), resulting in neonatal hypocalcaemia (< 2.0 mmol/L in term infants and < 1.75 mmol/L in pre-term infants). The incidence of hypocalcaemia is higher in mothers whose diabetes is less well controlled, especially in the third trimester. Hypocalcaemia is usually self-

limiting and very rarely presents with clinical signs. Expectant management is sensible and routine monitoring of plasma calcium is unnecessary.

## POLYCYTHAEMIA AND JAUNDICE

The mechanism for polycythaemia is thought to be the high cellular metabolic rate for glucose as a result of insulin-stimulated glucose entry, resulting in increased cellular oxygen uptake, relative hypoxaemia and stimulation of erythropoietin synthesis. This evidence comes from animal studies and also from human cordocentesis studies that have demonstrated that fetal blood lactate concentrations in the third trimester of diabetic pregnancies are higher than those of controls and are inversely proportional to blood partial pressures of oxygen.

Lysis of the large red cell load may explain the higher incidence of hyperbilirubinaemia and jaundice in the infants of diabetic mothers. In most infants, clinically significant sequelae do not result from the (usually mild) polycythaemia and hyperbilirubinaemia. If the haematocrit is greater than 70%, partial plasma exchange should be carried out.

## POSTNATAL CARE

All women with diabetes should be seen for a six-week postnatal examination. This consultation can be used to address a number of issues, including contraception. The progesterone-only (mini) pill has no significant effect on carbohydrate or lipid metabolism and can be safely used by women with diabetes both during breast feeding and in the long term. Modern low dose combined oral contraceptive preparations also have minimal effects on lipid and carbohydrate metabolism and can be used safely, especially in the younger woman. Sterilisation should be considered for the older woman who has completed her family.

For those who have had GDM, this consultation can be used to address a number of other important issues. First, these women should be offered a post partum OGTT to re-assess their glucose status. In the majority of cases this will have returned to normal. Arrangements can be made for follow up of those with established type 2 diabetes or IGT. Those who have reverted to a normoglycaemic status can be discharged to the primary care provider with the message that they are at high risk for the development of diabetes. This is greater in certain ethnic groups, e.g. women from the Asian sub-continent. Issues known to increase the time interval of normoglycaemia, such as maintaining a normal body mass index (BMI), reducing the fat content of the diet and increasing exercise, should be addressed. These women should also be advised to plan future pregnancies and encouraged to have a re-assessment of glucose status before conception.

## THE RISK OF DIABETES IN THE MOTHER FOLLOWING GDM

Incidences of diabetes between 3% and 65% have been reported in women who have had GDM. The incidence is greater the longer the follow up period after the index pregnancy. The risk of developing overt diabetes later in life is higher in women who develop GDM early in pregnancy. It is also higher in those who have had a significantly increased fasting plasma glucose concentration and in those who have been treated with insulin rather than diet alone. One of the best indicators for the future development of type 2 diabetes mellitus is an abnormal post partum glucose tolerance test. Other factors that have been shown to be predictive are the two hour glucose concentration or the area under the curve of the oral glucose tolerance test. Islet cell antibodies and insulin autoantibodies are well known predictive markers for type 1 diabetes. The presence of serum antibodies against glutamic acid decarboxylase (GAD65) has also been found to be an important predictor of type 1 diabetes. Because of the high risk of developing diabetes after the index pregnancy, regular assessment of glucose tolerance is important in women with previous GDM, to secure an early diagnosis of diabetes or impaired glucose tolerance.

## PREVENTION OF DIABETES IN THE MOTHER

The progression to diabetes following a pregnancy complicated by GDM is known to be influenced by both unmodifiable risk factors such as ethnicity, age and family history and potentially modifiable risk factors, which include obesity and future weight gain, physical activity and the composition of the diet. Preventative programmes need to focus on the modifiable risk factors. Obesity is the most important modifiable risk factor in the development of type 2 diabetes, as obesity and weight gain are important factors influencing insulin sensitivity. Weight loss in women improves insulin sensitivity, especially when associated with a decrease in abdominal fat distribution and waist-hip ratio. Significant metabolic improvement follows weight loss with improvements in glycaemia, lipid profiles and blood pressure. The evidence linking obesity with increasing risk of coronary heart disease in women provides further support for the case for readily accessible weight control programmes, especially in a group of women at increased risk of vascular disease from diabetes. All the evidence supports a policy that obese women with previous GDM should receive advice on weight loss and non-obese women on weight maintenance. It should then be emphasised that this is to delay the progression to diabetes as well as to reduce the risk of heart disease.

The prevalence of type 2 diabetes is highest in countries with a high fat intake and lower in those with a high carbohydrate intake. A high fat intake decreases insulin sensitivity and also increases the prevalence of other cardiovascular risk factors including hypertension, dyslipidaemia and obesity. Consequently, weight loss in women with previous GDM should be based on a decrease in dietary fat intake.

Physical activity is also important in primary prevention programmes. Physical activity promotes glucose uptake into muscle and increases insulin sensitivity. Regular physical activity helps to prevent increasing adiposity and reduces an individual's risk of developing type 2 diabetes. In addition to any benefits on carbohydrate metabolism, regular physical activity increases cardiovascular fitness and reduces cardiovascular risk factors including blood lipid concentrations, blood pressure and abdominal fat distribution. The recommendation of the British Heart Foundation is 20 minutes of activity three times per week, which can be achieved by brisk walking.

While definitive studies showing whether type 2 diabetes can be delayed or prevented are awaited, we should acknowledge that women with previous GDM are at heightened risk for both diabetes and cardiovascular disease and offer them the best advice on lifestyle behavioural modifications. They should, therefore, be counselled on the benefits of a low-fat diet, avoidance of obesity and the merits of regular exercise in addition to general advice on cardiovascular protection by blood pressure control, management of hypercholesterolaemia and cessation of smoking.

## RISK OF DIABETES FOR THE OFFSPRING FOLLOWING GDM

Diabetes begets diabetes, which should be expected as most major types of diabetes have a genetic basis. However, environmental influences such as the intrauterine environment are also thought to contribute to susceptibility. A diabetic intrauterine environment has a detrimental effect on adipocyte and pancreatic β cell development. The resulting effect on glucose metabolism may lead to the later development of type 2 diabetes. Most work on the development of diabetes in offspring of mothers with a genetic predisposition for diabetes has been in the Pima Indians. In this particular population, it has been shown that the diabetic intrauterine environment is a much more important determinant of type 2 diabetes than are genetic factors. The offspring of women with diabetes tend to be macrosomic at birth and are at increased risk of obesity in the future. This risk further contributes to susceptibility to diabetes.

Interestingly, there is now substantial evidence that poor fetal growth and low birth weight infants are also at increased risk for impaired glucose tolerance and diabetes in adulthood. This may be due to poor nutrition in fetal life, which is detrimental to the development and function of the β cells of the islets of Langerhans. It is suggested that this results in programming of metabolic pathways in the fetus resulting in insulin resistance.

Breast feeding may protect against type 1 diabetes through avoidance of exposure to cows' milk protein.

## FURTHER READING

Buchanan TA, Unterman TG, Metzger BE. The medical management of diabetes in pregnancy. Clin Perinatol 1985; **12**: 625-650.

Dornhorst A, Hadden DR. Diabetes and Pregnancy: An international approach to diagnosis and management, 1996. London: John Wiley & Sons.

Jovanovic-Petersen L, Peterson CM, Reed GF *et al*. Maternal postprandial glucose levels and infant birth weight: the Diabetes in Early Pregnancy Study Group. Am J Obstet Gynaecol 1991; **164**: 103-11.

Manning FA, Baskett TF, Morrison I, Lange IR. Fetal biophysical profile scoring: a prospective study in 1184 high risk patients. Am J Obstet Gynaecol 1981; **140**: 289-94.

Metzger BE Freinkel N. Accelerated starvation in pregnancy: Implications for dietary treatment of obesity and gestational diabetes mellitus. Biol Neonate 1987; **51**: 78-85.

Millner E, Hare JW, Cloherty JP *et al*. Elevated HbA1c in early pregnancy and major congenital anomalies in infants of diabetic mothers. N Engl J Med 1981; **304**: 1331-4.

Pedersen B. Hyperglycaemia-hyperinsulinism theory and birthweight, 1977. Baltimore: Williams and Wilkins.

Pedersen J. The pregnant diabetic and her newborn. Problems and management, 1967. Copenhagen: Munksgaard.

The Expert Committee on the Diagnosis and Classification of Diabetes Mellitus. Position statement. Diagnosis and classification of diabetes mellitus. Diabetes Care 2004; **27**: S5-S10.

Tulchinsky D, Little BA. Maternal–fetal Endocrinology, 1994. London: Harcourt Publishers Ltd.

# CLINICAL CASE

## GESTATIONAL DIABETES MELLITUS (GDM)

A 37 year old woman had had six pregnancies. Both her parents had type 2 diabetes.

The first two pregnancies were normal, resulting in the birth of healthy boys, both weighing over 3.6 kg. GDM was diagnosed in the second trimester of the third pregnancy. It was treated by diet but resulted in a stillbirth (3.92 kg) at 37 weeks.

GDM, again treated by diet alone, was a feature of pregnancies four and five, which resulted in the premature deliveries of a girl at 34 weeks (3.44 kg) and a boy at 32 weeks (2.53 kg), respectively.

The patient miscarried her 6th pregnancy and was subsequently diagnosed with type 2 diabetes. She was initially treated by diet alone. She became pregnant again a year later and was treated with insulin during the pregnancy.

Subsequently she has attended the Diabetes Centre regularly. She is obsese and her diabetes is difficult to control, with $HbA_{1c}$ values > 12.0%. She is currently receiving metformin and glicazide but is being persuaded to convert to treatment with insulin.

*POINTS:*

1.  GDM increases the risk of macrosomia and stillbirth.

2.  Women who have had GDM have a considerable risk of developing diabetes.

3.  Early delivery is often necessary in diabetic pregnancies, to ensure the health of the neonate.

4.  The effects of GDM are likely to be more severe in subsequent pregnancies to that in which it is diagnosed.

# Chapter 9

# Hypoglycaemia

## DEFINITION

A strict definition of hypoglycaemia is clearly of importance in identifying non-diabetic patients in whom further investigation is indicated. The commonly accepted blood glucose concentration below which hypoglycaemia is said to be present is 2.2 mmol/L. This is an arbitrary figure, owing much to the mg/dL figure of 40, rather than to any scientific approach. It should be appreciated that the definition is based on a venous or capillary sample although what is really important is the arterial glucose supply to the brain.

Systematic studies have shown that the lowest capillary blood glucose concentrations that occur in normal people are about 2.8 mmol/L. In normal elderly subjects (65 years or over) the lowest observed random blood glucose concentrations are around 2.5 mmol/L.

## HYPOGLYCAEMIA IN PATIENTS WITH DIABETES

In patients taking insulin, there is considerable variation in the concentration of blood glucose at which symptoms of hypoglycaemia develop, confirming that there is no one blood glucose concentration below which the patient is hypoglycaemic. The majority will not experience hypoglycaemic symptoms until blood glucose has fallen to concentrations generally accepted as indicating hypoglycaemia, that is, concentrations that trigger a counter-regulatory response. Some will experience symptoms suggestive of hypoglycaemia with blood glucose around 4.0 mmol/L, and occasionally patients claim to feel hypoglycaemic at relatively normal blood glucose concentrations.

The observation that some diabetic patients on insulin experience hypoglycaemia at normal blood glucose concentrations has led to the concept of relative hypoglycaemia. Hypoglycaemic symptoms at such times are suggested to be due to a rapid fall in blood glucose as a result of the action of insulin. It is suggested that a rapid fall from a concentration of 20 mmol/L to, say, 10 mmol/L may provoke symptoms by the speed of the fall. This may be relevant when the clinician has to decide whether bizarre symptoms in a patient taking insulin are due to the effects of hypoglycaemia. Some patients with diabetes claim that they like to maintain their blood glucose concentrations at around 10 mmol/L because at lower concentrations they feel unwell and hypoglycaemic. The traditional argument is that a patient used to running a blood glucose of 10 mmol/L or more may 'adapt' to this blood glucose concentration and feel hypoglycaemic at a lower concentration. It is uncertain whether there is any scientific basis to this explanation.

## PATHOPHYSIOLOGY OF HYPOGLYCAEMIA

The symptoms of hypoglycaemia are partly due to cerebral starvation of glucose (neuroglycopenic symptoms) and partly due to physiological responses (autonomic or neurogenic symptoms).

## CEREBRAL EFFECTS OF HYPOGLYCAEMIA

Glucose is the only readily available substrate supporting brain metabolism in man. Cerebral stores of glucose, as glycogen, are trivial, and therefore glucose must be transported via the blood from sources elsewhere in the body. Delivery of glucose to brain tissue is, therefore, not simply a function of blood glucose concentration but is also dependent upon cerebral blood flow. Entry of glucose into the brain is not normally a rate-limiting step and a reduction in glucose supply is followed by a decrease in intra-cerebral metabolism. It is this decrease that is of importance in stimulating the counter-regulatory response. The protective triggering of a counter-regulatory response by the brain seeks to obviate the consequences of hypoglycaemia on the brain, particularly the impact of cognitive dysfunction.

During prolonged fasting, the brain can adapt to use ketone bodies as energy substrates. However, this adaptive mechanism takes some time to develop and in normal daily living it has little or no role to play. A further adaptive mechanism may occur in the human brain when it is chronically deprived of glucose. This causes the counter-regulatory response to acute hypoglycaemia to occur at a lower blood glucose concentration.

## COUNTER-REGULATION

The release of the counter-regulatory hormones, glucagon, catecholamines, cortisol and growth hormone, is a survival response, the aim of which is to restore glucose supply to the brain. It involves the mobilisation of glucose from stores elsewhere in the body and transport to the brain via the circulation. Although all four of the major counter-regulatory hormones are capable of raising the blood glucose concentration, the mechanisms by which they achieve this and their specific functions within the response are different.

Adrenaline and glucagon promote glycogen phosphorylation, and hence glucose formation, in the liver. Growth hormone and adrenal corticosteroids have a more important role in prolonged hypoglycaemia through induction of gluconeogenic enzymes. While the initial responses raise blood glucose through mobilisation of glycogen, this is rapidly followed by an increase in gluconeogenesis. Catecholamines also increase rates of lipolysis and increase concentrations of circulating non-esterified fatty acids. These may decrease glucose uptake into muscle, making more available for uptake into the brain.

In recent years, great attention has been paid to defining the thresholds at which the various responses to hypoglycaemia occur. The sequence of events can be summarised thus: glucagon and adrenaline secretion occur when arterialised venous plasma glucose falls to 3.8 mmol/L; growth hormone secretion also occurs at around this concentration, but cortisol secretion requires a fall to 3.2 mmol/L. Symptoms are felt at 3.0 mmol/L and the onset of cognitive dysfunction occurs at around 2.7 mmol/L.

## ELECTROLYTE CHANGES
It is well recognised that the administration of insulin causes a fall in plasma inorganic phosphate concentration. This is likely to be a result of the entry of glucose into cells. Less well recognised is the fall in plasma potassium concentration during hypoglycaemia, which can produce ECG changes.

## CLINICAL ASPECTS OF HYPOGLYCAEMIA IN DIABETES
In clinical studies in diabetic patients, assessment of hypoglycaemia is often made and categorised into mild, symptomatic hypoglycaemia, with or without home blood glucose or laboratory glucose confirmation, and severe hypoglycaemia that requires third party assistance. It is probable that the frequency of hypoglycaemia in the diabetic population is underestimated by doctors, nurses, and even patients themselves. Asymptomatic hypoglycaemia in type 1 diabetic patients is common, particularly at night.

## CAUSES OF HYPOGLYCAEMIA
The concentration of glucose in the blood is determined by the amounts entering and leaving the blood. Reducing the amount entering the blood, increasing the amount leaving, or a combination of both, will lead to a fall in blood glucose concentration.

The most common cause of hypoglycaemia in patients with diabetes is delay or omission of a meal. Oral carbohydrate intake can be modified in advance if exercise is planned, but unplanned exercise may increase the risk of hypoglycaemia. The effect of alcohol is often difficult to predict. Most alcoholic drinks contain, or are mixed with, other drinks containing carbohydrate as sugar. Alcohol, however, inhibits hepatic gluconeogenesis and can therefore precipitate hypoglycaemia. Most people who experience an occasional hypoglycaemic attack are able to identify the reason for its occurrence. In a small group of patients, however, attacks develop a recurrent pattern, with or without any obvious cause.

## RECURRENT HYPOGLYCAEMIA

The majority of newly diagnosed type 1 diabetic patients retain the ability to secrete small amounts of insulin once over the acute hyperglycaemic stage. This remission or 'honeymoon' phase is usually fairly obvious. Once blood glucose has been brought under control, there is often a progressive reduction in the insulin requirement, starting within weeks and progressing over months. Home blood glucose monitoring results are in single figures and glycated protein concentrations are in the normal range. During this time, hypoglycaemia may be experienced unless proactive action is taken. The same is true of patients who are recovering from an infection, which has caused a temporary increase in insulin requirements.

Antibodies to injected insulin used to be a major cause of hypoglycaemia, particularly on changing a patient from a conventional (highly antigenic) beef insulin to a highly purified porcine or human insulin. This has ceased to be a major problem now that highly purified insulins are almost universally used.

Recurrent hypoglycaemia may occur with declining renal function. Although renal failure is associated with the development of insulin resistance, the predominant effect is a reduction in insulin requirements, which is presumed to be caused by reduced glucose production from renal gluconeogenesis and/or the increase in insulin's half-life in renal failure.

Endocrine disease resulting in reduced secretion of one or more of the counter-regulatory hormones may present as recurrent hypoglycaemia. This is common in Addison's disease but can also occur in hypopituitarism.

## SYMPTOMS

Symptoms of hypoglycaemia arise from the counter-regulatory responses, particularly the effects of catecholamines, and from cerebral starvation of glucose (neuroglycopenia). They consist of tremor, sweating, anxiety, hot and cold feelings, hunger, weakness and palpitations. Some patients experience a characteristic warning symptom of paraesthesiae around the lips and tongue. Headache and disturbance of vision are also common. Rarer symptoms include visual, auditory and olfactory hallucinations. Changes in mood and behaviour, particularly irritability, but also garrulousness, are often the earliest indication of an attack and the patient may fail to appreciate what is happening. If corrective treatment is not given, drowsiness and coma may follow.

## SIGNS

Sweating is probably the easiest sign to recognise. The brow is cold to the touch and there may be accompanying tremor and pallor. In the early stages, speech is often slurred. The picture may resemble that of acute alcoholic intoxication. All grades of disturbance of consciousness are possible from mild confusion to manic violence or deep coma. There is usually a rapid, bounding pulse as a result of adrenergic stimulation.

Occasionally, but well recognised, hypoglycaemia presents with focal neurological signs. Hemiplegia is quite common and it may be impossible to distinguish it from that caused by a stroke.

Chronic hypoglycaemia may also occur in patients with diabetes, usually as a consequence of over-treatment with insulin. Acute neuroglycopenic symptoms do not occur: it tends to present with behavioural change. When this occurs in elderly diabetic patients it may be confused with the deterioration in mental capacity that may be seen with cerebral atherosclerosis.

DIAGNOSIS

In most cases, the diagnosis is suspected from the fact that the patient is on insulin or oral hypoglycaemic drugs and that symptoms of mental confusion have appeared rapidly in someone apparently in good health. In normal daily life, most attacks are recognised by patients from the warning symptoms and signs with which they may be familiar. Treatment is given and the hypoglycaemic attack aborted. In more severe attacks, the patient may present to an Accident & Emergency Department with disturbance of consciousness ranging from confusion to coma. In this situation, the diagnosis should be confirmed by measuring blood glucose: it is extremely important to take a blood sample before giving any treatment. If it seems likely that the diagnosis is hypoglycaemia, treatment can be started immediately, without waiting for the laboratory measurement of glucose concentration. In the majority of occasions, when glucose promptly resuscitates the patient, the blood sample can then be discarded. It may prove invaluable, however, if there is a failure to respond. This is especially so in cases of prolonged hypoglycaemic coma, when recovery may be delayed for a considerable time.

If the blood glucose concentration is above 2.8 mmol/L, hypoglycaemia as a cause of unconsciousness is unlikely, although results may be confounded by the duration of the episode and any treatment given before the sample is taken.

Reagent strip tests should not be used to diagnose hypoglycaemia. In a deeply unconscious patient with well perfused peripheries it should be possible to obtain an adequate blood sample with which to confirm the result. More often, the patient is confused and perhaps aggressive: obtaining a blood sample may be difficult, and it may be tempting to collect only a capillary sample for reagent strip testing.

However, there is ample evidence that most reagent strip tests do not perform at their best when the blood glucose concentration is in the hypoglycaemic range. Disasters have been reported, and if measurement of blood glucose measurement is considered necessary, it should be a laboratory measurement on venous blood.

TREATMENT
Prevention is the best approach but when this fails, early intervention is appropriate. At the first symptom sugar, as glucose or sucrose, should be taken orally. A period of ten to fifteen minutes may be needed for recovery although, more usually, it is almost instantaneous.

Unconscious patients require intravenous glucose: 50 mL of 50% glucose will immediately raise the blood glucose concentration by at least 5.5 mmol/L. Injection of intravenous glucose at a concentration of 50% should be done with great care. The fluid is extremely viscous and, if extravasation occurs, extremely toxic to surrounding tissues. Subcutaneous or intramuscular glucagon (1 mg) is an alternative. Glucagon mobilises glycogen from the liver and its effect therefore is dependent upon glycogen stores and hence the nutritional status of the patient. In well nourished patients with adequate liver reserves, it will only raise blood glucose by approximately 2 mmol/L. It is considerably less effective in fasted patients. The effect may be enough to raise the conscious level sufficiently to allow oral intake but it should always be followed by oral carbohydrate. Intravenous glucose should be regarded as the first line of treatment, with glucagon being reserved for patients with difficult venous access.

In a few cases, recovery is slow or delayed despite treatment that raises blood glucose concentration. It is then particularly important to substantiate the diagnosis by measuring the blood glucose concentration in a sample taken before treatment. It is often difficult to explain why the patient fails to improve even though the blood glucose has been restored, although this is well recognised to occur.

IRREVERSIBLE BRAIN DAMAGE
Considering the large number of patients with diabetes who have major hypoglycaemic episodes, it is uncommon to see evidence of permanent brain damage. Focal neurological signs and even decerebrate posturing tend to resolve speedily with treatment. Delayed recovery from coma may take several days and yet seems to be complete in that the capacity to carry out exacting intellectual work is unimpaired.

FATALITIES
Death from hypoglycaemia is uncommon but not rare, accounting for about 3-4% of deaths occurring in young patients with diabetes. Many of the patients who die in this way have personality or psychiatric disorders.

The pathological changes found in the brain in fatal episodes are not specific and resemble those due to anoxic damage from any cause. There is widespread degeneration and necrosis of neurones with corresponding macroglial and microglial proliferation. The cortex, caudate nucleus and putamen are areas most severely affected; changes in the cerebellum and brain stem are less marked. Pathological changes can be difficult to interpret. Frequently, the terminal coma is prolonged and there is often associated severe hypoxia before reaching hospital. In addition the patient may need prolonged support of respiration and circulation on an Intensive Care Unit.

## SULPHONYLUREA-INDUCED HYPOGLYCAEMIA

A special mention must be made of the diabetic patient (or rarely a non-diabetic patient), who has a severe hypoglycaemic episode as a result of taking sulphonlyureas. It is common in Accident and Emergency Departments to see insulin-induced hypoglycaemia rapidly diagnosed and treated with a predictable regaining of consciousness in response to intravenous glucose. The patient can then be fed something more substantial and sent home. With sulphonylurea-induced hypoglycaemia, the initial response to treatment may be similarly impressive, but there remains a risk of recurrence of hypoglycaemia, making immediate discharge from hospital potentially dangerous.

This occurs because of the difference in the mechanism of hypoglycaemia induced by exogenous insulin and by sulphonylureas. A patient who is hypoglycaemic from sulphonylurea produces excessive amounts of endogenous insulin from the β-cells, which are 'primed' by the sulphonylurea to release insulin. The only tools for treatment of the low blood glucose are glucose or glucagon, both of which are insulin secretagogues. Thus the increase in blood glucose achieved by treatment is accompanied by a yet further increase in circulating insulin, making recurrent hypoglycaemia almost inevitable. Sulphonylurea-induced hypoglycaemia is a medical emergency that usually requires admission to hospital and careful monitoring of blood glucose concentrations to prevent relapse. Sulphonylurea-induced hypoglycaemia in a non-diabetic individual is discussed further below.

## NON-DIABETIC HYPOGLYCAEMIA

Hypoglycaemia occurring in non-diabetic patients requires careful investigation. The problem must be approached in a logical manner, since there is considerable scope for confusion and erroneous conclusion.

## THE HISTORY

Taking a history from a patient with possible symptoms of hypoglycaemia has two objectives. First, do the symptoms of which the patient complains bear any resemblance whatsoever to hypoglycaemic symptoms? And, second, if there is a possibility that the patient *is* experiencing hypoglycaemia, at what time of day is this occurring: in particular, do any of the attacks occur after an overnight fast? Fasting hypoglycaemia raises the distinct possibility of an insulin-secreting tumour, while hypoglycaemia during the rest of the day and particularly occurring 2-3 hours after a meal signals reactive hypoglycaemia.

DIAGNOSIS WHEN FASTING HYPOGLYCAEMIA IS SUSPECTED
Initial investigation involves taking fasting samples for measurement of glucose and insulin after three overnight fasts. If the glucose values are not in the hypoglycaemic range, the samples for insulin can be discarded, because under these circumstances the diagnosis is extremely unlikely and further investigation is usually unnecessary. If the history sounds convincing yet the three results are not diagnostic, more tests may be necessary. At this stage, a 72 hour fast may be performed. Some clinicians perform this as their initial investigation, but hospital admission is required to monitor the fast and collect samples if hypoglycaemia occurs. It is important that patients undergoing a 72 hour fast are not made to rest for the whole period. Glucose utilisation by muscle should be maintained by some exercise, possibly even vigorous exercise, although this may be poorly tolerated by someone who has fasted for more than 48 hours. On obtaining a fasting blood glucose result that is in the hypogly-caemic range, the sample for insulin that was taken at the same time should be sent for measurement of insulin and C-peptide.

Insulin assays have come under considerable scrutiny over the past few years. This followed the demonstration that most antibodies used in radioimmunoassays for insulin were non-specific, measuring proinsulin and proinsulin fragments in addi-tion to insulin itself. Immunoradiometric assays have now been developed that are specific for insulin; proinsulin and the split proinsulin derivatives, 31/32 and 63/64 proinsulins, can be measured in separate assays. Paradoxically, it does not help in the diagnosis of insulinoma to measure insulin specifically. The tumours may be either predominantly insulin or proinsulin secreting. This partly explains why a patient may be seen with only a modest lowering of blood glucose but a high (non-specific) insulin concentration that is due mainly to proinsulin reacting in the radioim-munoassay for insulin. In the investigation of a possible insulinoma, it is best to measure 'insulin' using a non-specific radioimmunoassay.

Unfortunately, doing this can complicate interpretation of the results. Clearly, the concentration of insulin measured will reflect the specificity of the antibody. Thus it is likely that different laboratories will obtain different values for insulin concentra-tions although, it is to be hoped, similar values for blood glucose. This being so, it is not possible to specify a ratio of glucose to insulin that will be diagnostic of an insuli-noma; as a result, the diagnosis depends simply upon the presence of hypoglycaemia not suppressing insulin secretion appropriately and the concentration of insulin being raised out of proportion to the concentration of glucose.

The use of stimulation and suppression tests to confirm the diagnosis has fallen out of favour. Stimulation tests were always somewhat inappropriate, contrary to the adage that oversecretion of a hormone is diagnosed by a suppression test and under-secretion by a stimulation test. For stimulation, glucose, tolbutamide, leucine and glucagon have been employed. For this purpose, they range from useless (glucose) to dangerous (tolbutamide). Of the suppression tests that have been used, adrenaline did not prove useful and only fish insulin provided the basis for a useful test. Fish insulin was given to lower blood glucose to a concentration that in a normal person would inhibit endogenous insulin secretion. Provided samples were assayed using an antibody that did not react with fish insulin, inhibition or failure of inhibition of secretion could be detected.

In the vast majority of patients with an insulinoma (up to 95%) the diagnosis is made from one of three fasting glucose and insulin samples. A few more will be diagnosed by proceeding to a 72 hour fast when there is a high index of suspicion. The next question is whether to attempt pre-operative localisation of the tumour. Although ultrasound, CT scanning, coeliac axis angiography and MRI scanning have all been used, opinions differ on their usefulness. All would agree, however, on the importance of an experienced surgeon used to searching for the tumour by palpation of the pancreas.

Wherever possible, treatment is surgical. Medical treatment is by inhibition of insulin secretion with diazoxide, usually combined with hydrochlorthiazide to counteract the side-effect of fluid retention. Medical treatment is usually limited by an inadequate response, fluid retention or the growth of unsightly hair over the whole body.

Insulinomas may be multiple, particularly when the hyperinsulinism is part of the syndrome of multiple endocrine neoplasia (MEN) type 1. Tumours are malignant in about 5% of patients, almost always with detectable secondary spread to the liver.

OTHER CAUSES OF FASTING HYPOGLYCAEMIA
Other endocrine disease such as Addison's or hypopituitarism may present with fasting hypoglycaemia due to reduced secretion of one or more of the counter-regulatory hormones, which have actions antagonistic to insulin.

In the fasting state, the maintenance of blood glucose concentration is heavily dependent upon hepatic glucose output and extensive liver disease may result in hypoglycaemia. End stage renal failure is associated with insulin resistance yet there is also a risk of hypoglycaemia. In part this is due to the loss of renal gluconeogenesis, which may be particularly important in mildly acidaemic patients. It may also reflect reduced insulin clearance.

REACTIVE HYPOGLYCAEMIA

Reactive hypoglycaemia is undoubtedly a real condition, although the incidence is difficult to estimate owing to lack of diagnostic rigour. At times, the diagnostic label has been evoked to explain behaviour that might be better labelled bizarre or frankly psychopathic, but more usually it has been used to explain symptoms of hunger, lethargy and lassitude that might conceivably originate from a low glucose concentration. In certain populations, it has been a fashionable complaint at times, generating an industry in its management (if not its diagnosis). The confusion arises because of ignorance over the glucose tolerance test. In normal subjects we are used to seeing two hour glucose tolerance tests with a rapid rise in blood glucose concentrations after oral glucose and a return to fasting concentrations by two hours. If these tests are extended for five hours, there is a fall in blood glucose below the baseline at around three hours, frequently followed by a gradual return to normal. In some normal subjects, calculating the area under the glucose curve over five hours will even give a negative value, that is, the area below the baseline from 2-5 hours is greater than the area above the baseline from 0-2 hours. It must be stressed that this is a normal finding and a fall in blood glucose at three hours to 3.5 mmol/L is *not* diagnostic of reactive hypoglycaemia.

In a few patients, this fall is exaggerated, and a blood glucose concentration of 2.2 mmol/L is reached and accompanied by symptoms compatible with hypoglycaemia. These people may be regarded as normal, that is, they have no underlying pathology, yet they have symptoms that are uncomfortable and, in certain situations, are disabling or even dangerous, and they therefore deserve advice and treatment. The glucose tolerance test, however, delivers a non-physiological load of rapidly assimilated carbohydrate and even if a fall in glucose concentration occurs that is sufficient to warrant the label of hypoglycaemia in the absence of symptoms, there remains a concern as to the relevance of this to everyday life when carbohydrate is taken as a variety of simple and complex sugars.

This glucose tolerance test response is thought to come about by a rapid insulin secretory response, which rapidly dissipates the glucose in the blood, after which insulin concentration is inappropriately high. It certainly is true that symptoms are more likely to occur if highly sweetened drinks are taken. Occasionally, this exaggerated pattern of the glucose tolerance test may be a prodrome of type 2 diabetes.

There is never any point in measuring insulin in suspected reactive hypoglycaemia and, indeed, it can be argued that in investigating hypoglycaemia there is never any point in measuring insulin in any other than the fasting state. Ignoring this advice can lead to the generation of potentially misleading data and (avoidable) difficulties in diagnosis.

## FACTITIOUS HYPOGLYCAEMIA

Factitious hypoglycaemia occurs when insulin or a sulphonylurea is taken deliberately by a patient, or administered deliberately by a third party. In either situation, the condition is extremely difficult to diagnose. Hypoglycaemia may be obvious and lead to investigation for insulinoma. Often it is only when all possible diagnoses are ruled out that the suspicion of factitious hypoglycaemia crosses the mind. Certain pointers in the history may help but they can also mislead. Anecdotally, it has been suggested that the majority of patients with this condition are from the medical or allied professions, particularly nursing or pharmacy, yet insulinomas also occur in patients in these professions. It is equally as likely that these patients may be mislabelled as having factitious hypoglycaemia as having an insulinoma.

On suspecting the diagnosis and confirming hypoglycaemia with hyperinsulinism, the first question is whether the hyperinsulinism is endogenous or exogenous. The answer to this question is given by measurement of C-peptide. If the hyperinsulinism is endogenous, C-peptide will be co-secreted and its concentration raised; if exogenous, endogenous insulin and C-peptide will be suppressed by the hypoglycaemia. When insulin and C-peptide are both raised, it is worth screening the sample for the presence of a sulphonylurea, which can be performed in specialist centres. If C-peptide is suppressed, an alternative approach must be employed. Confrontation is rarely successful and alternative approaches, such as searching the patient's belongings, may be illegal. Searching a hospital room or ward toilets is not illegal and occasionally reveals the heights of imagination and deviousness that patients may scale to hide supplies of insulin and syringes.

FURTHER READING

Amiel SA, Sherwin RS, Simonson DC, Tamborlane WV. Effect of intensive insulin therapy on glycaemic thresholds for counter-regulatory hormone release. Diabetes 1998; **37**: 901-7.

Clark PM. Assays for insulin, proinsulin(s) and C-peptide. Ann Clin Biochem 1999; **36:** 541-64.

DCCT Research Group. Epidemiology of severe hypoglycemia in the Diabetes Control and Complications Trial. Am J Med 1991; **90:** 450-9.

Heller SR, Cryer PE. Reduced neuroendocrine and symptomatic responses to subsequent hypoglycemia after one episode of hypoglycemia in nondiabetic humans. Diabetes 1991; **40**: 223-6.

Marks V, Teale JD. Investigation of hypoglycaemia. Clin Endocrinol (Oxf) 1996; **44:** 133-6.

Marks V, Teale JD. Hypoglycaemia: factitious and felonious. Endocrinol Metab Clin North Am 1999; **28:** 579-601.

Mitrakou A, Ryan C, Venemen T *et al*. Hierarchy of glycaemic thresholds for counter regulatory hormone secretion, symptoms and cerebral dysfunction. Am J Physiol 1991; **260:** E67-E74.

Owen OD, Morgan AP, Kemp HG *et al*. Brain metabolism during fasting. J Clin Invest 1967; **46:** 1589-95.

# CLINICAL CASES

## INVESTIGATION OF HYPOGLYCAEMIA

A 20 year old electrician complained to his family doctor of recent onset of episodes of dizziness lasting for 10-20 minutes. There did not appear to be any precipitating factors. He had experienced these episodes mainly in the afternoon; none had occurred before breakfast. He was otherwise well and was not taking any prescription medication. His mother had type 1 diabetes and while symptomatic with one of these episodes he had tested his blood glucose on his mother's home blood glucose meter, which had recorded a result of 2.5 mmol/L. He was very muscular in appearance and was an amateur weight-lifter although there was no recent weight gain. He denied taking steroids.

On examination he weighed 94 kg, height 172 cm, BMI 31.8 kg/m$^2$. Blood pressure was 110/70 mmHg. Neurological examination was normal. He was referred to a consultant diabetologist for investigation for suspected insulinoma.

Three consecutive overnight (16 hour) fasts failed to produce hypoglycaemia (morning venous plasma glucose concentrations being 5.2 mmol/L, 5.0 mmol/L and 4.8 mmol/L, respectively). A prolonged oral glucose tolerance test was performed:

| Time (min) | Plasma glucose (mmol/L) |
|:---:|:---:|
| 0 | 4.9 |
| 30 | 5.2 |
| 60 | 9.7 |
| 90 | 8.5 |
| 120 | 7.7 |
| 150 | 3.9 |
| 180 | 3.0 |
| 210 | 3.0 |
| 240 | 4.5 |
| 270 | 5.0 |
| 300 | 4.7 |

The patient was followed up regularly in out-patients for a period of six months. He remained well and did not experience any further episodes.

*POINTS*

1.  In the history it is important to attempt to ascertain whether episodes suggestive of hypoglycaemia are occurring mainly fasting or in the post absorptive state. Where there is no clear history of episodes occurring before breakfast, a 5 hour glucose tolerance test may occasionally be helpful, and be a more appropriate investigation than searching for fasting hypoglycaemia.

2.  During a prolonged OGTT, a fall in plasma glucose concentration to a level below that recorded for the fasting sample is seen in normal individuals 3-4 hours into the test. However, plasma glucose concentrations do not normally fall to levels that would cause neuroglycopaenic symptoms ( $\sim < 2.5$ mmol/L ).

3.  Up to 95% of patients with an insulinoma experience hypoglycaemia during one of three overnight fasts.

4.  A possible explanation for these episodes could be steroid or insulin abuse. Both are recognised causes of hypoglycaemia in weight-lifters and body-builders. Insulin abuse by body-builders is probably on the increase and should be considered in young people who 'work out' in a gym and present in an Accident & Emergency Department with symptoms of hypoglycaemia.

## FACTITIOUS HYPOGLYCAEMIA

A 19 year old student nurse complained to her family doctor of 'dizzy spells', having had three such episodes in the previous month. These took the form of sudden onset of light-headedness, tremor and sweating, lasting for a few minutes. Two of these episodes had occurred whilst at work and had been relieved by sitting down and drinking a cup of coffee (two spoonfuls of sugar). On the second of these occasions, a capillary blood glucose of 2.8 mmol/L was recorded on the ward blood glucose meter.

No abnormalities were found on clinical examination. Initial laboratory investigation including urea, electrolytes and full blood count were normal, and a urinary pregnancy test (beta-HCG) was negative.

Following referral to an endocrinologist, three overnight fasts on consecutive nights were performed for the investigation of insulinoma. The corresponding morning plasma glucose concentrations were 5.2 mmol/L, 4.2 mmol/L and 4.3 mmol/L.

While awaiting follow up, she experienced a further episode at work and was taken to an Accident & Emergency Department. A blood glucose of 2.1 mmol/L was recorded on the A&E Department blood glucose meter. A glucose sample analysed in the laboratory confirmed hypoglycaemia, with a plasma glucose of 1.8 mmol/L. The senior house officer also took samples for insulin and C-peptide, which were immediately transported to the laboratory on ice. The patient was treated with intra-venous 50% glucose and made a full recovery.

Laboratory results from admission :

| Analyte | Result | Reference range (fasting) |
|---|---|---|
| Plasma | | |
| Glucose (mmol/L) | 1.8 | |
| Insulin (pmol/L) | 85 | < 35 |
| C-peptide (pmol/L) | 183 | 370 ± 30 |

The low C-peptide concentration was inconsistent with the high insulin concentration, indicating that the insulin was largely exogenous. The patient later admitted self-administering insulin and was treated for anxiety and depression.

*POINTS*

1. Three consecutive overnight (16 hour) fasts result in hypoglycaemia, with non-suppressed insulin levels, in up to 95 % of cases of insulinoma. Further investigations include prolonged fasting (72 hours), accompanied by exercise if necessary.

2. Factitious hypoglycaemia should be considered, particularly where the patient has access to insulin or sulphonylurea, e.g. in a healthcare worker, or carer or relative of a patient with diabetes.

3. Differentiation between insulinoma and factitious hypoglycaemia is by measurement of insulin and C-peptide at the time of hypoglycaemia. Insulin and C-peptide concentrations cannot be interpreted if the patient is not hypoglycaemic (plasma glucose < 2.2 mmol/L). Samples for insulin and C-peptide must be collected on ice and transferred immediately to the laboratory for centrifugation.

4. Glucose results measured by near patient testing blood glucose meters are less reliable at the upper and lower extremes and abnormal results must be confirmed by measurement in the laboratory.

# Index

## U

UK Joint Working Group on Quality Assurance guidelines for point of care testing in DM, 122-123

United Kingdom Prospective Diabetes Study (UKPDS), 51, 64, 99, 113, 116

## V

Viruses and type 1 DM, 2

## W

West of Scotland Coronary Prevention Study (WOSCOPS), 104

WHO diagnostic criteria for DM, 38

WHO recommendations for diagnosis of gestational diabetes, 132-133

WHO recommendations for glucose measurement, 37

NOTES